The
BIOMECHANICALLY
CORRECT TRAINING SYSTEM

The thinking person's guide
to unilateral resistance training

DARREN VARTIKIAN

TOH
Triangle of Health
Publishing

First published 2013 by Triangle of Health Publishing
PO Box 707, Wentworthville, NSW 2145, Australia.
www.triangleofhealth.com.au

Typeset in Times New Roman 11/13.5 pt
Copyright © 2013 Darren Vartikian
The moral rights of the author have been asserted.

National Library of Australia Cataloguing-in-publication data

Author:	Vartikian, Darren, author, illustrator.
Title:	The biomechanically correct training system: the thinking person's guide to unilateral resistance training / Darren Vartikian; editor Maggy Saldais.
ISBN:	978-0-9875690-0-4 (paperback)
Notes:	Includes bibliographical references.
Subjects:	Isometric exercise.
	Exercise.
Other contributors:	Saldais, Maggy, editor.
Dewey number:	613.7149

Cover design and internal design: Pipeline Design (www.pipelinedesign.com.au)
Illustrations and photographs: Darren Vartikian
Editor and proofreader: Maggy Saldais
Licensed images provided by: Dreamstime (www.dreamstime.com)

9 8 7 6 5 4 3 2 1

To my friends Dr Joseph Azize, Chiropractor Sam Dona and Brett McCarthy:
thank you for your input, encouragement and support
during the evolution of this book.

...

Special thanks to my editor Maggy Saldais and designer Peter Reardon:
you promised me something special and you delivered. You gave me more than
money could buy – you actually cared. What a team!

This book is dedicated to all people who are passionate about:

- *resistance training, health, fitness and well-being*
- *illness prevention*
- *alleviation of frustrating and debilitating injuries*
- *increasing athletic performance.*

CONTENTS

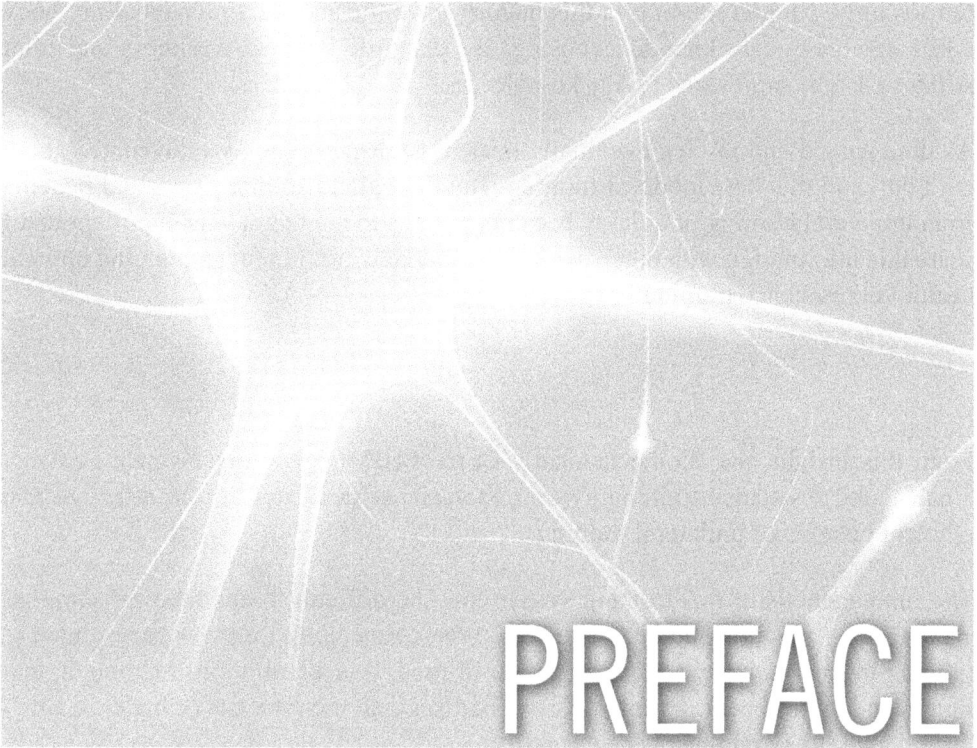

PREFACE

I truly believe that everything happens for a reason and that every cloud has a silver lining. In 2004, my 'cloud' was an uncharacteristic pain in the front upper left thigh. I dismissed it as a training-related issue that would go away in time. Months passed and the pain persisted, becoming ever more painful.

After I had consulted multiple physicians and had numerous X-rays and scans, an osteoid osteoma, a benign bone tumour, was diagnosed. Radio frequency ablation was the treatment and surgery was scheduled for early 2005. The procedure would allow me to go home the next day, signifying the start of the recovery process and the resumption of a normal life.

Resuming training in the gym two weeks after surgery, I found myself restricted not only with lower body exercises, but also with those for the upper body. Like most people in the gym, I then employed traditional bilateral resistance training: contracting and exercising muscles on either side of the body at the same time.

My disability impeded such training so I had to adapt accordingly. I realised that I needed to carry out all my exercises in a unilateral fashion, exercising one muscle on one side of the body at one time. For the first time in all the years I had till then been involved in resistance training, I started using unilateral training for the whole body.

Surprisingly, I found training in this manner gave me an awareness about my body I had not previously known, exposing, for example, muscle weakness and joint stiffness. I felt empowered by the knowledge.

As time passed and my leg eventually healed, I felt increasingly rejuvenated about my body and this new mode of training. Having gained so many personal benefits from unilateral training, it quickly became obvious to me that it was important that I share this information with others who had a shared commitment to attaining optimal health via resistance training.

. . .

From this insight, the Biomechanically Correct (BMC) Training System evolved, a calculated resistance training system exclusively dedicated to the effective and efficient benefits of unilateral training.

The fundamentals of this training system may be difficult to embrace for some, as change can be daunting and habits hard to break, especially for those accustomed to training in a certain way for a long period of time. It is a reality of life, though, that illness and injury occur. Eventually, one realises – in the interests of better health – that change (to avoid these) is a necessity.

I have tried to break the BMC Training System down in a way that is simple and easy to follow, removing the frustration that can come with learning something new.

'I am not endorsing change for the sake of change, but for
the betterment of the mind and body.'

INTRODUCTION

T he Biomechanically Correct Training System: the thinking person's guide to unilateral resistance training is a comprehensive guide to resistance training that involves exercising one muscle on one side of the body at one time.

This system – analytical, calculated, meticulous, systematic and user-friendly – dares to be different in its approach to resistance exercise.

The book has four easy-to-use sections:

- *Section One* explains what resistance training is and its benefits, and the various methods and equipment that can be used.

- *Section Two* dissects the nature of unilateral resistance training. It explains why it is an imperative training regime for anyone concerned about safety, maintaining structural integrity to avoid injury, and developing muscles at an optimal level, while allowing affected joints to move in the most efficient way. The section also broadly analyses some of the problems and risks associated with traditional bilateral resistance training.

- *Section Three* breaks down the components of unilateral training – addressing issues such as position, direction and motion – and answers questions pivotal to achieving safe and maximum performance from muscle and exercise. By way of contrast, it also provides further reasons why common compound exercises for resistance training should be avoided.

- *Section Four* outlines various prime moving muscles, describing their position and function, and unique associated exercises that best develop, strengthen and condition them individually.

Whether you are a novice or have years of experience with resistance training as a form of exercise, it is important that this book is read from cover to cover. This will eliminate any potential confusion about the *how*, *what*, *where* and *why* of the various aspects of this training system – referred to hereafter as the BMC Training System.

Ultimately, the main objective of this book is to guide, educate and enlighten readers about the many benefits of unilateral resistance training.

'You can say it and know it – but it doesn't matter unless you do it.'

SECTION ONE

Biomechanically Correct Resistance Training

People who use resistance training as a form of exercise generally set out to achieve their goals with great passion and conviction. Unfortunately, most do so without first having a calculated structure and organisation that provides direction, guidance and a rationale for what they are doing.

Learning anything new can be a simultaneously exciting and anxious experience. The BMC Training System endeavours to remove the daunting aspects of learning new things, providing easy-to-understand guidance on unilateral resistance training exercise.

It outlines what to do so results are achieved with minimal risk of injury, and provides clear guidance on how to execute unilateral resistance exercises. It also describes the logic for why some things are encouraged and others discouraged.

. . .

Who will benefit from the BMC Training System? The answer is almost everyone (qualified because anyone under the age of 18, with mental or physical disadvantage, or with lack of experience in resistance training should **not** attempt the exercises except under the supervision of an exercise professional). This system is inclusive and will allay many fears some might have about weightlifting (e.g. that it will make women muscle bound).

The BMC Training System is a unique resistance training system dedicated to achieving goals in a safe, efficient and productive manner. It has been developed through applying theory, as well as practical knowledge and experiences learned about the human body.

To appreciate the true value of this training system, knowledge of the various components of resistance training, and its relationship with the human body, is required.

'Don't judge it until you try it.'

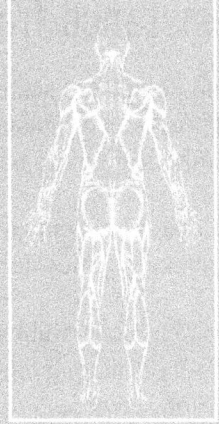

1
What is Resistance Training?

Just as a car needs servicing, so, too, does the human body. Our bodies are sophisticated pieces of machinery made up of subsystems. One subsystem, catering to physical activity, is the musculoskeletal system; it consists of the skeletal and muscular systems. Resistance training is an essential means of strengthening and conditioning the musculoskeletal system and increasing the body's longevity.

So what is resistance training? It is a form of exercise whereby the weight or load of equipment, such as barbells or dumbbells, creates resistance against a contracting muscle with subsequent movement of weight in a push-or-pull manner.

Resistance training is a form of anaerobic exercise; that is, physical activity carried out by energy produced in the absence of oxygen.

Resistance training, or weight training as it is also known, is the foundation of sports such as bodybuilding, powerlifting and weight lifting, and is an important adjunct to other sports as a means of increasing power, strength and skeletal muscle size.

'Resistance training exercise is paramount for optimal health and fitness.'

Resistance Training Fears

Some people are scared of resistance training as a form of exercise; others deem it inappropriate or make excuses to avoid attempting it. Some of these fears are valid, but others are quite unfounded.

One fear, prevalent among women and athletes in some sports, is that lifting weights will make you muscle bound, decreasing agility and effectively disrupting movement.

A common oversight with this type of thinking is that resistance training is only one component among other variables (such as nutrition) that will dictate or limit desired goals or outcomes.

Another deterrent influencing some people's thinking – and that has some legitimacy – is simply a lack of knowledge.

Without knowledge, it is easy to be deterred from trying something new. Resistance training is no exception. Not knowing how to use a piece of equipment or carry out an exercise can be daunting. The opposite can also be true: too much information can confuse, disillusion and frustrate. Enlisting the help of an exercise professional in a health and fitness facility, together with proactive reading and research, is highly recommended for the novice individual.

Intimidation is another reason why some people avoid resistance training. Training facilities and gyms, certain individuals and some equipment can all be potentially intimidating. Sometimes this is unintentionally the case – for example, some women may find it uncomfortable, or intimidating, simply sharing a fitness environment with the opposite sex. Fortunately, this issue is easily remedied: women can join a women-only gym or one that is segregated.

The sight of certain resistance training equipment can also overwhelm some people, raising genuine fears of injury. Injury is certainly always a possibility when equipment is used incorrectly or contrary to its intended purpose, or when an individual lacks focus. The intention of this book is to provide the necessary instruction and guidance so this does not happen.

...

Resistance training as a form of exercise and to achieve goals should be viewed as a lifelong objective. The following three ingredients are paramount for success:

1. *Encouragement:* This helps to keep the fires of motivation alive. This encouragement can come from yourself; your family, friends, instructors and trainers (coaches); and from the general staff at health and fitness facilities.

2. *Patience:* Take your time and enjoy the experience! Don't be in hurry. Taking your time and being consistent will give you the best results in the long term.

3. *Realistic expectations:* Above all, do not set the bar too high. This will avoid feeling overwhelmed or disappointed.

Benefits of Resistance Training

As technology continues to develop rapidly, so, too, does the convenience with which daily tasks are carried out. Unfortunately, this benefit comes with a price: decreased levels of physical activity, which ultimately affect health, fitness and well-being.

Muscles of the body perform four important functions:

1. *Movement:* Muscles contract creating propulsion and locomotion via the joints.

2. *Energy storage:* Energy is stored in the form of glycogen within muscles.

3. *Protection:* Muscles create protective barriers for organs of the body.

4. *Stability:* Muscles help to preserve the structural integrity of the skeletal system.

Any weakness or deterioration from disuse will guarantee a decline in the function of the muscular system, creating a domino effect for the skeletal and nervous systems. This will ultimately lead to malfunction and poor health.

The saying 'use it or lose it' is an appropriate way to describe the importance of resistance training. The benefits for skeletal muscles from resistance training occur as a result of the following linear process:

1. Resistance training creates a weight or load to which a muscle is unaccustomed.

2. This training breaks down muscle fibres.

3. Provided that a person has sufficient nutrient consumption and rest, muscle healing and adaptation then occur.

4. This, in turn, creates a stronger, better conditioned and more efficient functioning muscle.

Therapies such as physiotherapy, chiropractic, osteopathy, massage, kinesiology and psychology have evolved to rehabilitate, heal and resolve issues of a physical and mental nature. Resistance training should be viewed in the same way.

'Iron therapy' – using resistance equipment – expedites healing of injuries and assists in the relief of stress and anxiety-related issues, reducing reliance on other therapies for structural maintenance.

There is also the issue of optimal muscle function – and, yes, appearance, too. In a world obsessed with appearance, the past two decades have seen the ageing process become big business. Turn on a TV, listen to the radio or jump onto the Internet and you will find a commercial or advertisement endorsing a cream, lotion, potion, nutritional supplement or device that will supposedly reverse or slow down the ageing process, revitalising youthful appearance. Cosmetic procedures such as botox and collagen injections, liposuction and surgeries have also flourished to combat the ageing process.

There is no doubt that procedures such as plastic surgery can tighten sagging skin, and botox injections can eliminate wrinkles (even if temporarily); unfortunately, both remedies fall short as a long-term solution. The end results are temporary in their efficacy, and do not address the real issues associated with the ageing process.

Unfortunately, with age, muscle tissue decreases and so does its ability to function efficiently.

The most obvious way of gauging the ageing process is the extent of wrinkling or sagging of skin, both side effects of muscle atrophy.

Either through ignorance or an obsession to achieve a youthful appearance, people often lose sight of the obvious solution: muscle tone is the key. Increasing or maintaining the integrity of muscle tissue guarantees muscle tone, ensuring tighter, firmer looking skin. This is best achieved through weight-bearing resistance.

Below are a few examples of health benefits that resistance training offers (by increasing or maintaining the size, strength and conditioning of skeletal muscles):

- It ensures that joint and connective tissue are properly aligned, reducing degeneration, subsequent aches and pains and energy expenditure.

- It maintains the protective housing environment for organs, and the efficient function of blood and nerve vessels, subsequently allowing muscle contraction, digestive processes, hormone production and other chemical reactions to function at an optimal level.

- It ensures the effective and efficient use of body fat for energy, via the furnace-like component of a muscle cell called the mitochondria.

- It reduces tension, bringing about a state of relaxation, while increasing flexibility and unrestricted movement.

- It promotes healing of the mind, body and spirit.

A lack (or neglect of) resistance exercise in the long term will only result in muscle atrophy and a decrease in both strength and bone density, ultimately leading to poor health.

Who Benefits from Resistance Training?

Everyone can benefit from resistance training, be they male or female, adult or child, exercise novice or professional athlete.

Resistance Training for Athletes

Athletes all around the world, at all levels, are always looking for that 'added edge' in their chosen sport. The answer is resistance training. It is the perfect adjunct to any sport, working as a tool to increase athletic performance.

So, how can resistance training help with your chosen sport? Simple!

Consider the responses to these three questions:

1. What do all sports involve?

    Answer: Movement.

2. What creates movement?

    Answer: Muscles and joints.

3. What develops, strengthens and conditions muscles and joints?

    Answer: Resistance training exercise.

However, there is a note of caution: it is essential that athletes keep in mind that imitating movement patterns of certain sports with weighted resistance can be dangerous.

Resistance training should be looked upon primarily as a way of developing the body, not used as a mimicking tool for a chosen sport.

The benefits of resistance training generally become evident in the following order:

1. *Feeling:* increases in energy levels, well-being, happiness and optimism
2. *Function:* increases in power, strength and endurance
3. *Appearance:* changes to physical structure, increased tone, decreased body fat and greater muscle definition.

Aside from the obvious health benefits, resistance training can also be an immense source of relaxation – a way to release stress and to make time for reflection and solitude away from the pressures and demands of everyday living.

Resistance Training for Children

The suggestion that children should engage in resistance exercise may shock some; there may be concern that a child's normal growth and development would be impeded and/or damaged.

The argument against resistance training as a form of exercise for children is founded around two main issues:

1. *Intensity:* The amount of effort used during a resistance exercise is a legitimate source of concern, especially when a heavy, inappropriate weight is used.

2. *Incorrect exercise technique:* This will cause problems whether one is a child, an adult new to resistance training or an elite athlete. Executing a resistance exercise incorrectly over time will lead to poor muscle development and increase the likelihood of structural damage (to varying degrees).

With these potentially negative aspects acknowledged, it's important to realise that there are, nonetheless, legitimate benefits for children from resistance training.

Resistance exercise teaches a child discipline, structure and commitment, while increasing the strength, health and development of the child's mind, body and self-esteem. If parents are to embrace resistance exercise as an integral part of a child's life, any stigma (in respect to its perceived associated danger) needs to be removed. That being said, this does not mean that parents should not fully inform themselves of inherent risks before starting. It is also critical that any child under 18 undertaking a program of resistance training be closely supervised by an established exercise professional.

Ultimately, undertaking resistance exercise safely and productively - for children, or anyone - is achieved by emphasising and implementing the proper technique.

Focusing on executing an exercise correctly, without worrying about load or intensity, is *paramount* and plays a pivotal role in the BMC Training System. This makes it the perfect resistance training system for children.

Products of Resistance Training

The simultaneous contraction and interaction of a muscle and object produces an energy called force. It is force that allows the movement of an object.

In resistance training there are three ways to measure force: power, strength and endurance. Each represents a measurement of muscle force through an allocated number of muscle contractions known as repetitions. Repetitions performed during an exercise will dictate the type of force produced.

- *Power* is the force created through a combination of strength and speed that muscles produce within a short number of explosive contractions. Muscle power can be developed with repetitions ranging from 1 to 6.

- *Strength* is the force muscles produce within a moderate number of muscle contractions. Muscle strength can be developed with repetitions ranging from 8 to 12.

- *Endurance* is the force muscles produce during a sustained number of muscle contractions over a period of time. Muscle endurance can be developed with repetitions greater than 13.

Each repetition range will produce a specific outcome relating to hypertrophy, strength or increased aerobic capacity (Table 1.1).

Table 1.1: Products of resistance training.

FORCE	TIME PERIOD	NO. OF REPETITIONS	PRODUCT
Power	Short	1 to 6	Explosive power
Strength	Moderate	8 to 12	Strength/Hypertrophy
Endurance	Sustained	13+	Muscle endurance

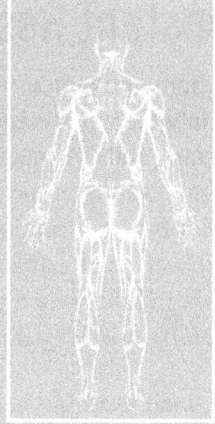

2
Methods of Resistance Training

T here are five methods of resistance training, each carried out with a specific muscle contraction and speed. Each method may or may not require joint movement, associated equipment or a unique mechanism for creating resistance and/or affecting movement speed.

The various equipment and mechanisms for resistance and movement encompass pin- or plate-loaded machines that may incorporate a lever, cam, cable-pulley, hydraulic or compressed air system; free weights, such as barbells and dumbbells; or the simple use of body weight.

As well as having a choice of resistance training methods, one can also choose between multi- and single-joint training.

'Knowledge empowers people to make correct decisions.'

Constant Resistance Training

Constant resistance training, executed through an isotonic muscle contraction, is one in which the resistance weight of the equipment used during an exercise remains constant and unchanged from beginning to end of the muscle contraction. Body weight exercises such as push-ups, chin-ups and crunches are the simplest form of this type of training, as are any exercises that use equipment such as barbells, dumbbells and cable-pulley machines. The disadvantage of constant resistance training is that when a muscle begins to fatigue, it loses musculoskeletal leverage, generally mid-way through a contraction.

One such example is the biceps barbell curl (Figure 2.1); when the biceps become fatigued, the weight will become much more difficult to move mid-way through the exercise.

Figure 2.1 Barbell curl

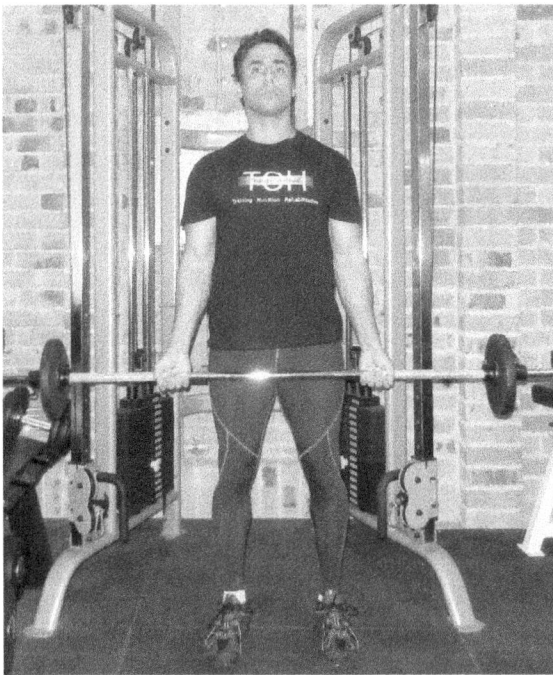

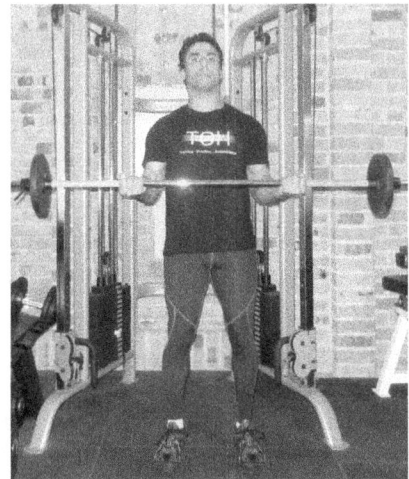

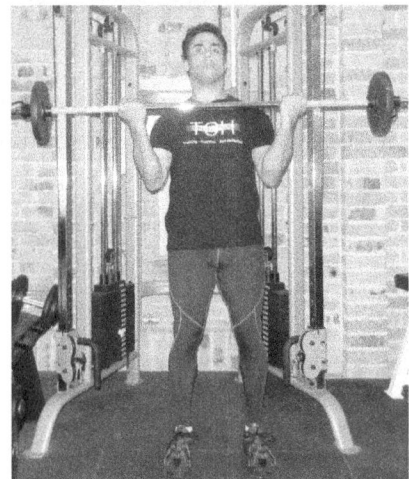

Variable Resistance Training

Variable resistance training, executed with an isotonic muscle contraction, is one in which the resistance weight of the equipment used during an exercise changes during muscle contraction.

The resistance weight will increase or decrease with an increase or decrease of musculoskeletal leverage, created through devices such as a cam, elliptical pulley or rolling lever arm.

The positive aspect of variable resistance training is the ability to overcome the leverage disadvantage of constant resistance training; the negative aspect is that it is impossible to cross-match every person and machine for optimal function.

Accommodating Resistance Training

Accommodating resistance training is a form of isokinetic exercise, executed with an isotonic muscle contraction.

Isokinetic exercise requires the use of specialty equipment in which the mechanism for resistance, either hydraulic or compressed air, functions to control muscle contraction and movement of the apparatus at a constant, controlled velocity or speed.

The theoretical advantage of isokinetic exercise is that, by maintaining movement at a constant speed, leverage is maintained; this allows a muscle to complete a contraction from beginning to end unaffected.

Unfortunately, accommodating resistance training is unnatural, as muscles contract in an accelerated and decelerated manner, not at a constant speed.

Plyometric Resistance Training

Plyometric resistance training – created in a rapid, explosive fashion using body weight (Figure 2.2) or weight-bearing equipment such as a medicine ball – focuses on the eccentric phase of an isotonic muscle contraction.

Due to its explosive nature, plyometric resistance training is not an appropriate form of resistance exercise for developing the size and strength of a muscle.

(*Note:* Carrying out plyometric resistance training can increase the risk of injury, if underlying structural problems go unnoticed.)

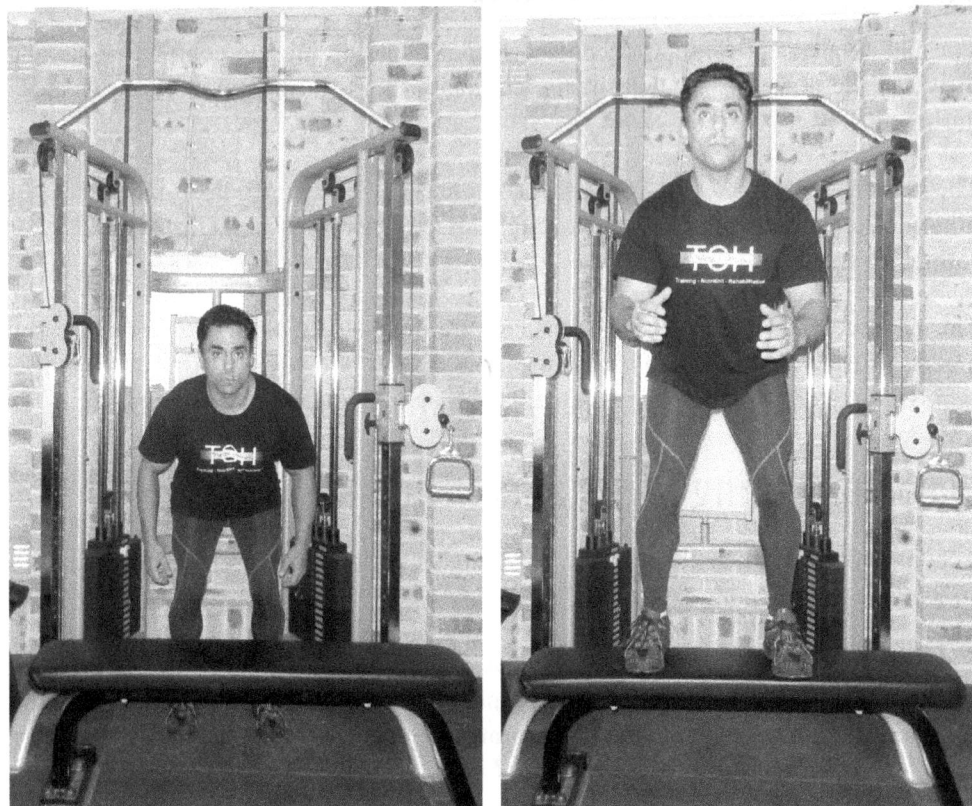

Static Resistance Training

Static resistance training is a form of isometric exercise executed with an isometric muscle contraction. It involves placing a muscle against an immovable object, followed by a gentle push or pull action for a nominated period of time. This creates a muscle contraction without joint movement (Figure 2.3).

Some people will regard static resistance training as a boring exercise, exacerbated by the fact that – to develop the size, strength and condition of a muscle completely – multiple positions and angles are necessary. This makes static resistance training a time-consuming 'chore' for some people.

However, static resistance training can be advantageous for rehabilitation and as a diagnostic tool to pinpoint muscle weaknesses, noticeable as muscle shaking.

Figure 2.3 Push and pull for the chest and trapezius muscles

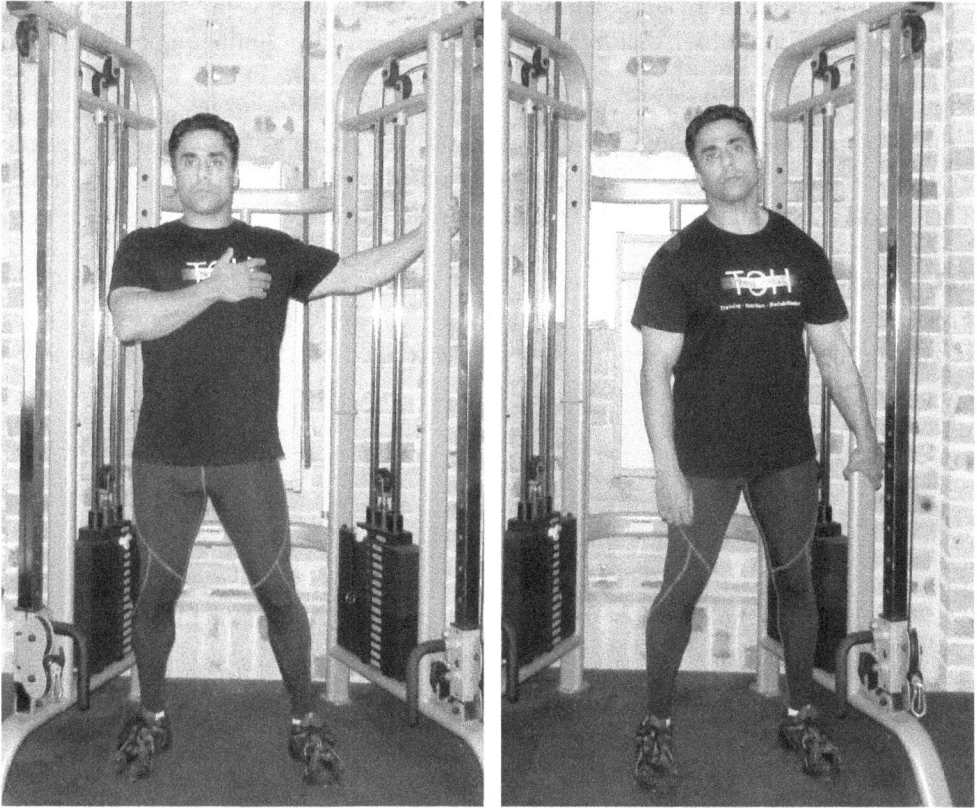

Multi- and Single-joint Exercises

Any form of resistance training exercise that uses multiple joints and muscles is commonly referred to as a compound exercise. The appeal and benefit of such an exercise is exercising multiple muscles at the one time; this allows use of greater weight, expediting muscle growth, strength and conditioning. Although good in theory, a compound exercise has some major flaws (discussed in more detail in chapter 12):

* It limits the isolation and analysis of a prime moving muscle, decreasing awareness of muscle weaknesses and increasing the potential for injury.

* It results in poor distribution of resistance through a prime moving muscle, increasing the likelihood of long-term muscle imbalance.

* It requires an increased expenditure of energy, unnecessarily exhausting the body as a whole.

An example of a compound exercise is the barbell squat (Figure 2.4), recognised as one that develops the quadriceps. Its movement involves the hip, knee and ankle joints, using muscles of the lower back and hips, the quadriceps and the hamstrings to name a few.

Any form of resistance training that uses a single joint and muscle action is commonly referred to as an isolation exercise. An isolation exercise is the closest possible means of totally isolating a prime moving muscle, eliminating other muscle assistance.

With less peripheral muscle involvement, greater focus is placed on the prime moving muscle, allowing optimal development of size, strength and conditioning. This is something that unilateral training caters to perfectly.

The 'opposite' of a compound exercise (for example, the barbell squat shown in Figure 2.4) is the leg extension (Figure 2.5), an exercise that isolates the knee joint and quadricep muscle and is generally executed on (but not limited to) a leg extension machine.

Figure 2.4 Barbell squat

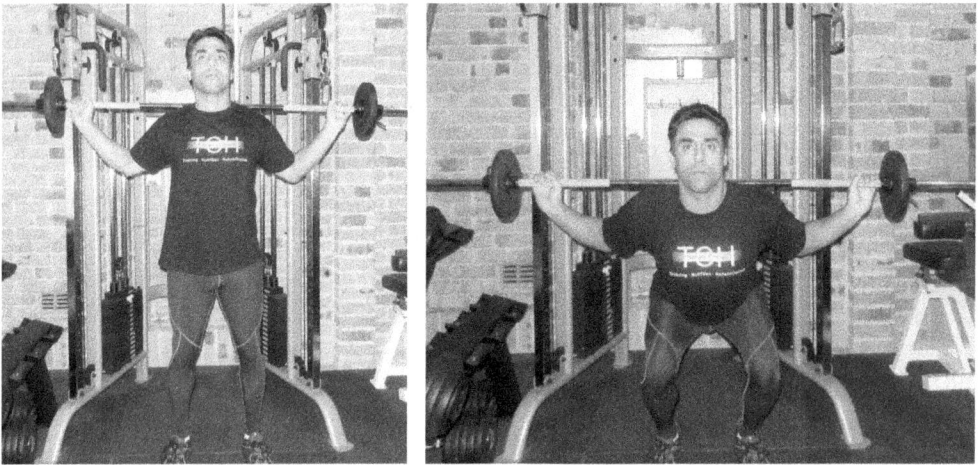

Figure 2.5 Leg extension

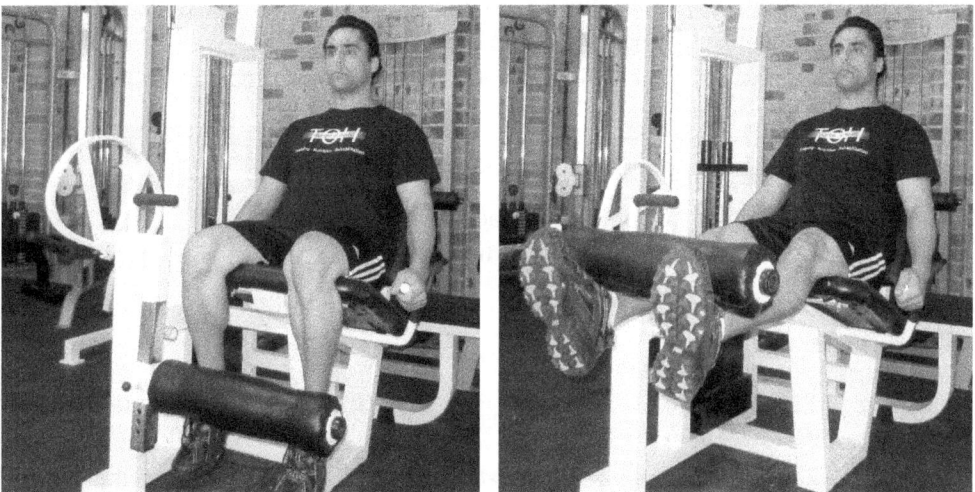

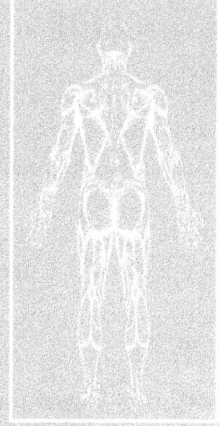

3
Resistance Training Equipment

The evolution of the health and fitness industry, like every other human endeavour, is a constant progression, though not necessarily always for the better. Every year, companies roll out the latest in resistance training equipment, claiming it to be the best in the hope of capturing a slice of the exercise market.

On offer for the consumer are various brand lines, machines for specific body parts, and pin- or plate-loaded machines with features such as range limiting devices and other adjustable points. The consumer then has the daunting task of sifting through the jargon and 'hard sell' of marketing brochures and campaigns to find what is most appropriate and safe to use.

It is only human nature that people constantly seek and desire something different, especially if it makes life easier and delivers results faster. But shopping for resistance exercise equipment – or deciding which health and fitness facility to join – should be dictated by productivity and safety, not by aesthetics, cost saving or convenience.

It is for these reasons, when one is considering buying or using a piece of resistance equipment, that one should give utmost importance to ensuring that it matches (in its function) the natural biomechanics of the human body.

'Think before you leap.'

Free Weight

A free weight, which is used to execute constant resistance training, can be a piece of equipment or apparatus that provides a weight or load that is not fixed to any structure and moves freely.

The most common and widely recognised free weights found in any gym worldwide are the barbell and dumbbell (Figure 3.1).

Barbell

A barbell is a straight bar, generally made of metal, that allows the placement of discs on each end, known as weight plates; these create the actual weight.

There are three types of barbell:

- *adjustable barbells*, which allow the convenience of placing and removing weight plates; these are generally found in home gyms

- *fixed barbells*, which have weight plates secured through welding or screws

- *Olympic barbells*, much larger than a standard barbell, which cater to lifting large amounts of weight. These are used during powerlifting and Olympic weight-lifting competitions.

Dumbbell

The dumbbell is a miniature version of a barbell and generally comes in a set of two; hence, it is commonly referred to as a pair of dumbbells.

There are three types of dumbbell:

- *adjustable dumbbells*, which allow the convenience of removing and replacing weight plates (although this can become tedious and annoying after a while)

- *fixed dumbbells*, much like the barbell, which are secured either through welding or special screws, making them safer and easier to use; these are found generally in commercial gym environments

- *moulded dumbbells*, which come as one solid piece, without any adjustable or removable components; these are generally made from solid cast iron, or cast iron covered with soft vinyl, and are useful in class or group fitness settings.

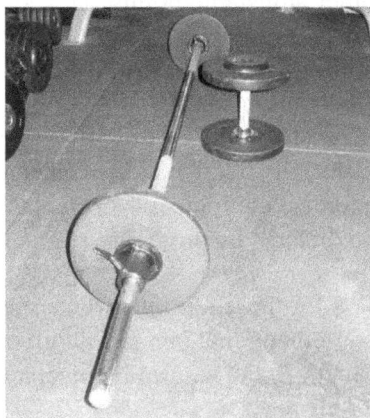

Figure 3.1 Barbell *(left)* and dumbbell

Machines

Resistance machines function through various systems, mechanisms or devices. Some are pin-loaded, with the weight in a stack of plates being changed by placing a metal pin into the hole of a weight plate; the weight then moves up and down steel rod shafts. Other machines are plate-loaded, with weight plates or discs being placed onto the fixed metal sleeve of a machine.

Cable-pulley

The cable-pulley system is the simplest form of resistance machine used in executing constant resistance training. It is made up of the following components: pulley, cable, weight stack, guide rods and structural frame.

Metal wire enclosed in a plastic sheath creates the cable, which is placed through a round fixed plastic or steel structure known as a pulley. The function of the pulley is to guide and support the cable, which is used to lift the weight that creates the resistance.

One end of the cable is secured to a weight stack, made up of individual weight plates; the other loop-shaped end functions as an attachment point for various bars or handles. Cable-pulley machines can be either single purpose (with fixed pulleys, designed to cater to one specific movement and muscle group) or multifunctional (Figure 3.2) (equipped with rotating and adjustable pulleys that accommodate optimal muscle contraction by allowing changes in position, height, angle and plane).

Nautilus

Nautilus machines are a brand of exercise equipment that incorporates a device known as a cam (which caters to variable resistance training). A spiral-like structure, the cam, much like a pulley, has either a cable or rubber belt attached to it, functioning to create efficient movement of the machine's weight.

The concept behind the cam system is as follows: it provides varying resistance, corresponding with the strength of a prime moving muscle, by bypassing the point of mechanical disadvantage, so that a muscle contracts, without inhibition, through a full range of motion. A cam will change the load of a weight at the weakest point of a muscle contraction without change to the amount of weight lifted.

Lever

Lever machines incorporate a lever system catering to variable resistance training, whereby movement of weight is created through a fulcrum and lever. When force is applied to a lever arm in a pull-or-push manner, the roller (which functions as the fulcrum) allows movement along the lever arm and the subsequent raising of weight attached to the machine.

Hammer Strength

Hammer strength machines are plate-loaded machines catering to variable resistance training that attempts to match the natural biomechanics of the human body.

The moveable arms have been developed to allow movement in a unilateral fashion, though not exclusively, creating resistance for each limb independently. Hammer strength machines create movement in a fixed converging and diverging manner.

Hydraulic

Hydraulic machines are specialty pieces of equipment that cater to accommodating resistance training by controlling and maintaining a constant speed of motion.

The mechanism for controlling movement speed is fluid inside a cylinder, guaranteeing mechanical leverage from beginning to end of a muscle contraction.

(*Note:* Ballistic, explosive movements using hydraulic machines are impossible to carry out.)

Figure 3.2 Multifunction cable-pulley machine

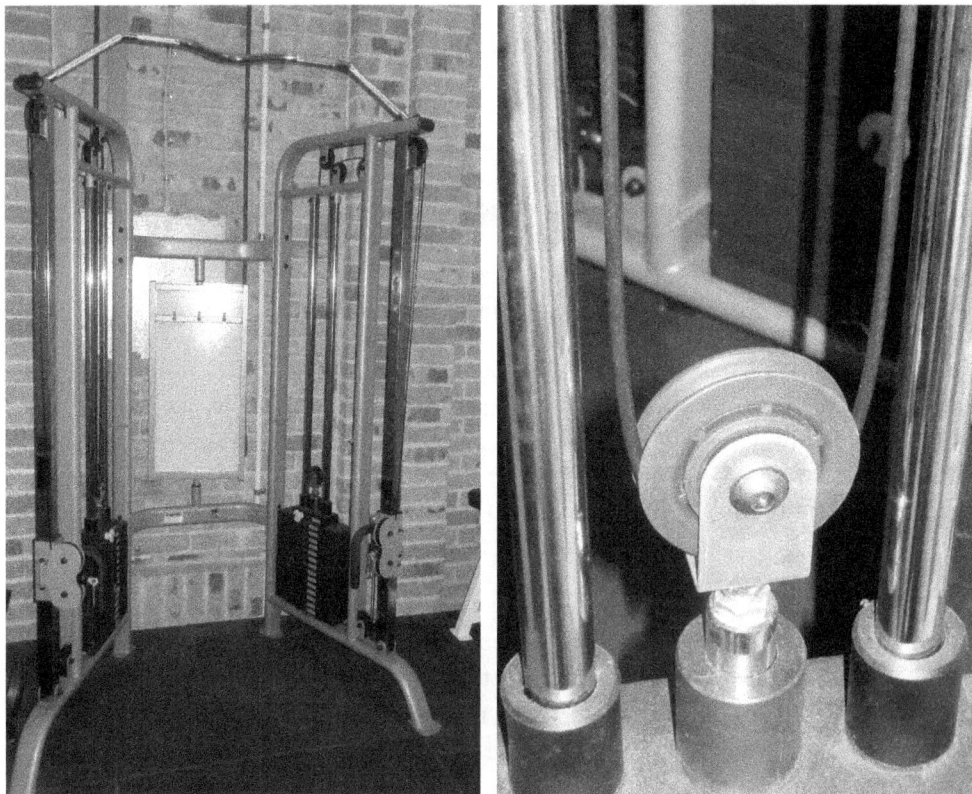

Static Devices

Static devices are immoveable objects used to execute static resistance training. A static device can be any object, apparatus or machine against which a muscle is placed to carry out an isometric muscle contraction in a push or pull manner (Figure 2.3) for a nominated period of time.

Body Weight

The human body is the simplest form of resistance training equipment. It can be used to execute constant resistance exercise, using body weight to perform a chin-up (Figure 3.3), push-up (Figure 3.4), sit-up (see pages 157–8) and various other exercises.

Figure 3.3 Chin-up

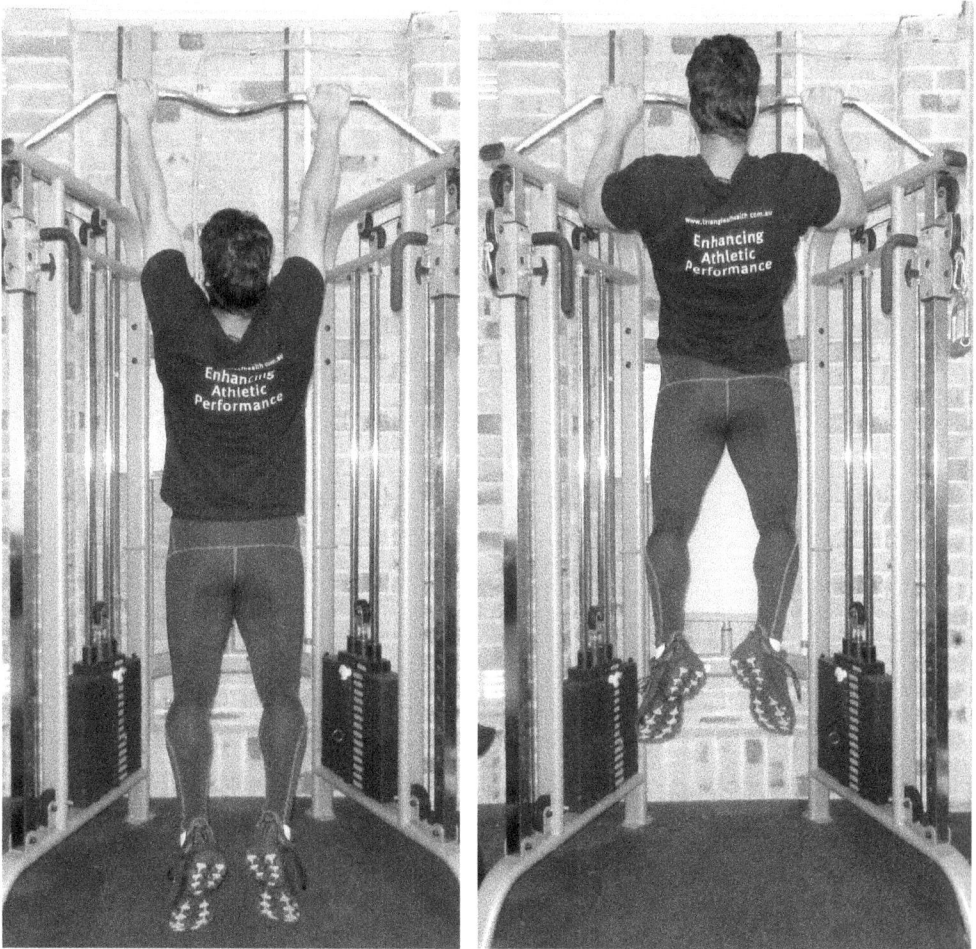

Figure 3.4 Push-up

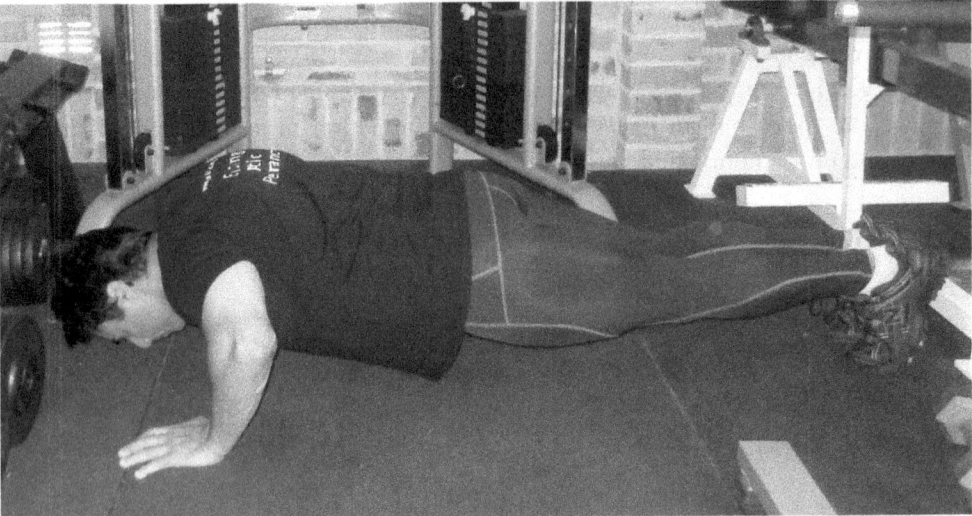

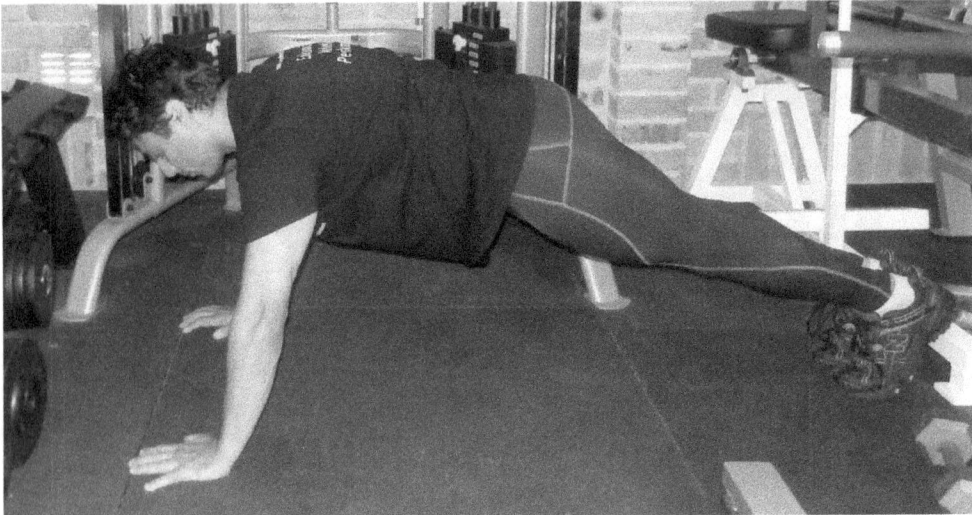

SECTION TWO

BMC Training System
Foundation

In Section One, the benefits, various methods and different types of equipment associated with resistance training were outlined. Section Two focuses on the most appropriate and efficient way to use resistance training exercise for maximum benefit.

All bilateral muscles of the body function independently. In many instances, they do so during everyday activities such as walking, running, swimming, writing, eating and so on, when using one limb at a time.

Recognising, therefore, what is already a natural process of independent function, the BMC Training System is built on the view that all resistance training should be executed in a unilateral fashion – *one side and one muscle at a time*. Unilateral resistance training allows a prime moving muscle to function in its most natural path of movement, accurately coordinating body parts to capitalise on leverage and balance, so that replication of precise biomechanics can be attained for maximum results and safety during an exercise.

This type of training is highly advantageous during instances when a prime moving muscle may execute more than one action or function, allowing the corresponding muscle on the other side of the body to work independently and efficiently, without competition or compromise.

Everyone, be they male or female, young or old, elite athlete or resistance training novice, can reap the benefits that unilateral resistance training has to offer.

For example, unilateral resistance training is an ideal way to introduce the elderly to resistance exercise, as it comes without the stigma of intimidation often associated with traditional bilateral resistance training – such as a fear that lifting a weight may harm or injure. It is also useful in rehabilitation after injury, providing essential, direct and specific control of muscle movement.

Unilateral resistance training defies any perception that resistance exercise is a time-consuming, boring chore that will only cause acute or chronic injury.

(*Note:* No matter what the goal, the end result of any form of resistance training exercise should be about creating and maintaining a healthy state of mind and body.

The body is designed so that its natural warning system of malfunction will activate – as pain, swelling and discomfort – if inappropriate resistance exercise is executed. Ignoring the warning system's signals will ultimately lead to varying degrees of short- and long-term structural damage.)

'The ideal resistance exercise uses resistance equipment that caters to the natural function(s) and biomechanics of a prime moving muscle so as to facilitate maximum benefit and minimal risk of injury.'

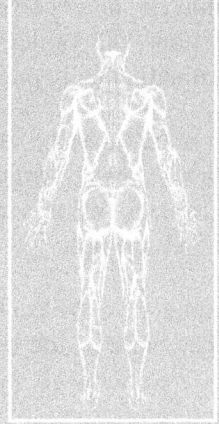

4
Unilateral Training

Unilateral resistance training offers many and varied benefits. The most valuable benefit, however, compared with traditional bilateral resistance exercise, is awareness. Awareness includes knowledge about the strength or weakness, and overall function, of a prime moving muscle. This insight allows precise analysis, empowering an individual with information about related issues and areas of the body, and expediting assessment and comparison.

Unilateral training transfers complete ownership of a resistance weight used during an exercise exclusively onto a single prime moving muscle, heightening the need for greater focus, which in turn decreases the contribution from accelerated momentum.

The reason why some injuries can occur in striving to develop balanced muscles is accelerated momentum. This generally occurs as a result of muscle exhaustion, imbalance in muscle strength, poor mental focus or just plain ego. A classic example of accelerated momentum is as follows: an individual executing a barbell curl with too much weight begins to generate movement through the hips, back and shoulders to raise the weight, instead of the intended prime moving biceps muscles. Unilateral training keeps the prime moving muscle 'honest': it eliminates the lifting of unrealistic amounts of weight and places limbs, joints and muscles in the best possible leverage position so that optimal strength during an exercise can be attained.

A muscle may carry out multiple actions, necessitating movement in varied directions and angles. Unilateral training accommodates this perfectly, accurately coordinating body parts free of restriction for optimal function and injury reduction.

That same versatility enables a prime moving muscle to be isolated during an exercise so as to precisely target a contraction of aspects that relate to the upper, lower, outer and inner fibres; this increases the potential for complete development of a muscle's size and strength.

Symmetry, in the context of resistance training, means that the muscles either side of the centre of the body are similar in appearance (size and shape) and function. They are effectively mirror images of each other, thus improving overall balance and structural integrity of the body. Barring genetic factors, unilateral training enables superior muscle development.

Time is a precious commodity most cannot afford to waste, making unilateral training the ideal form of resistance training for those with a busy lifestyle. A unique aspect of unilateral training is the allotted time of a workout. At face value, unilateral training might seem time-consuming; in fact, the opposite is true. The isolating nature of this type of training means reduced resistance weight which, in turn, decreases the exhaustion of the body as a whole. This enables faster recovery, and shorter rest periods between sets and exercises, resulting in a reduced workout time.

Prevention of injuries is a critical and integral feature of unilateral training. This goal is achieved by distributing resistance weight and muscle-generated force through a natural movement pattern, which protects muscle, joints and connective tissue.

Another element of injury prevention and balanced muscle development are motor units. A single motor neuron that connects to skeletal muscle fibres is referred to as a motor unit; it is the communication link between the brain and skeletal muscle, enabling muscular contraction. Skeletal muscles are made up of multiple motor units, making varied movement patterns a necessity, so that the total contraction and stimulation of a prime moving muscle occurs. This guarantees proper development. Unilateral training is the appropriate method to achieve this objective.

Relying on another person to assist during a workout can be very frustrating. A time to meet has to be coordinated, and the other person needs to turn up on time. An even greater concern for many is asking for assistance from someone they don't know; there may be concern, for instance, about the individual's level of experience with resistance training exercise.

Exercising one limb at a time affords the opportunity, circumstances permitting, of using the opposing limb (or other limbs not being used to assist during an exercise); this eliminates the burdensome need to rely on others.

'The facts are undeniable.'

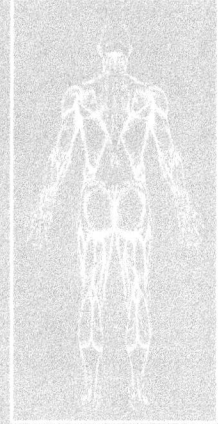

5
Negative Effects of Bilateral Training

Traditionally, resistance training exercise is executed in a bilateral fashion using nominated corresponding prime moving muscles on either side of the body. The barbell bench press, barbell deadlift and barbell biceps curl are just a few examples of common bilateral exercises. (See Chapter 12 for more detailed information on the negative aspects of these compound exercises.) There is no doubt that bilateral training is a very fast way of achieving muscle size, power and strength. Unfortunately, the desired results can also cause collateral damage – structural injuries to muscles, joints, connective tissue and nerve fibres. There is also the financial burden to rectify related injuries (medical and therapeutic practitioner costs) and the psychological frustration due to physical pain or exercise restriction, which can be long term.

One way to describe the potential risks of bilateral training is to compare it to someone using a shotgun for target practice. Many pellets or bearings encased in the bullets would be dispersed during the shooter's attempts to hit the bullseye, causing unintended damage to the rest of the target in the process (Figure 5.1).

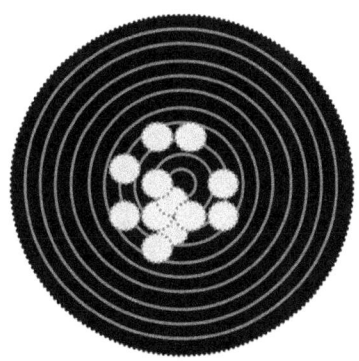

Figure 5.1 Collateral damage of hitting the bullseye

Damage to the body (whether short-or long-term) – in the form of soft tissue tears and strains, bone degeneration or general aches and pains caused as a result of bilateral training – results from one of two things:

- repetitive strain to the muscles, joints and connective tissues
- an imbalance of muscle development or strength and conditioning that each ultimately relate to inappropriate and inefficient movement patterns.

Exercising muscles bilaterally increases the compensatory effect, hampering one's awareness and eliminating the ability to correctly analyse strength, weakness and the injury potential of corresponding muscles either side of the body (Figure 5.2).

Figure 5.2 Muscle weakness compensation during a barbell biceps curl

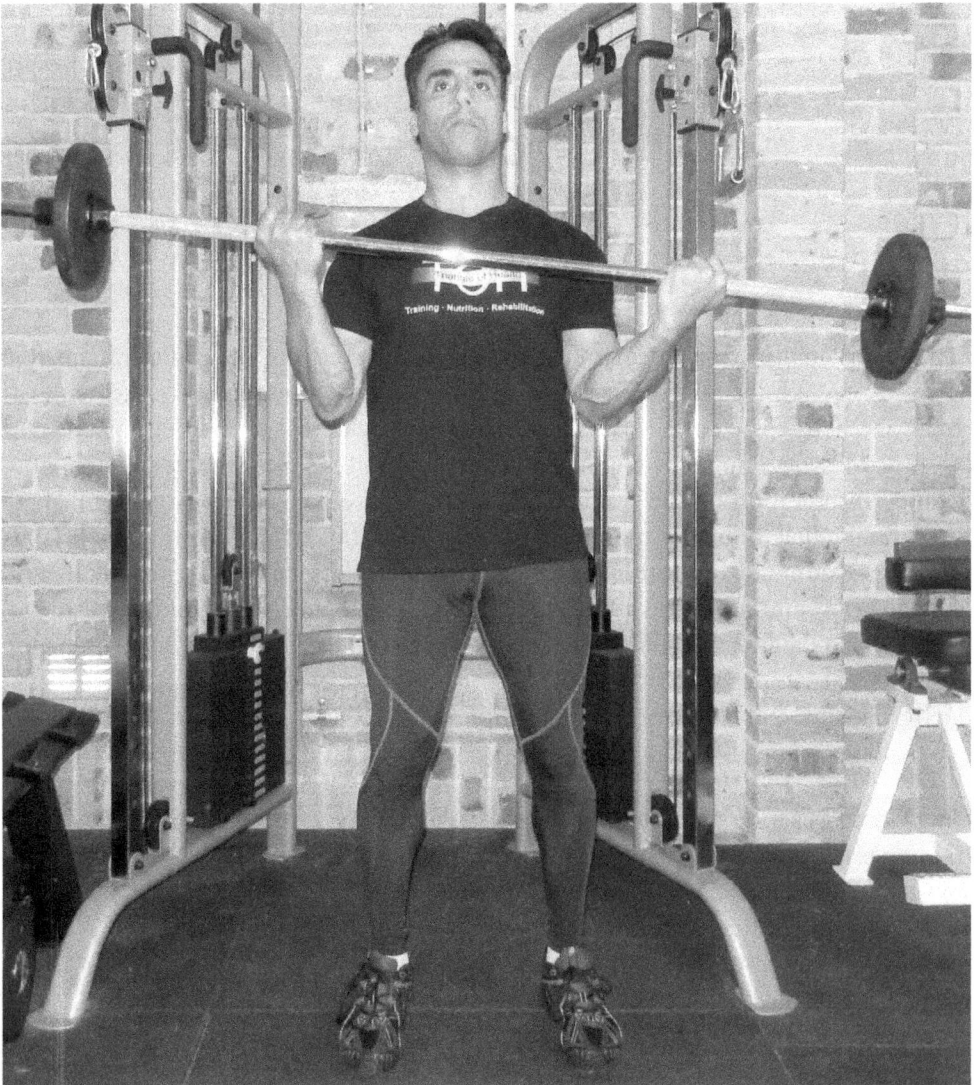

There is no disputing that bilateral training enables an individual to lift a greater amount of weight, resulting in quick gains in size, power and strength. Unfortunately, this can also have negative consequences:

- It can lead to the formation of dangerous weight-lifting habits, such as using accelerated momentum (through bouncing, swinging or thrusting of a weight) to try to overcome mechanical disadvantage. Moving a weight using accelerated momentum bypasses two of the body's natural protective mechanisms – muscle spindles and golgi tendon organs – increasing the risk of injury.

- It increases the potential for hyper-stimulation of the nervous system, increasing the risk of exhaustion or burn out to the body as a whole and necessitating the need for more rest. Consequently, progress is slowed.

- Lifting greater weight increases training intensity, energy expenditure and the length of rest periods, making movement between sets and exercises slow. This leads to longer time spent working out.

- The need for a safety net (in the form of a spotter) is synonymous with bilateral training. Lifting heavy weights necessitates having someone close by in case help is required. This means either having to rely on a training partner or constantly having to ask someone for help (which may annoy the person asked).

'Just because everyone is doing it, does not mean it is right.'

SECTION THREE

Components of Unilateral Training

B eing interested in resistance training as a form of exercise is one thing; maintaining that interest is another. To help sustain motivation, confidence and enthusiasm, some knowledge of and guidance in resistance training are imperative.

Section Two outlined unilateral training as the fundamental basis for the BMC Training System. Training one muscle on one side of the body at a time is just one aspect of this training system.

Another important aspect – and, indeed, a key goal – of the BMC Training System is creating a structured process that teaches an individual how to exercise muscles and associated structures in the most natural, efficient and effective manner possible.

To achieve this, the following key components of unilateral resistance training need to be explained:

- prime moving muscle, divided into sections for exercise

- ideal position of the body and associated structures for exercise

- movement pattern, the path of contraction for a prime moving muscle

- inertia, overcoming the stumbling block for a muscle contraction

- speed, volume and intensity, relating to muscle and exercise

- equipment – the most effective for unilateral resistance training.

Analysis of each of these components in subsequent chapters of Section Three has evolved through trial and testing, producing a structured, user-friendly training system.

'The BMC Training System is about exercising muscles,
not exhausting the mind and body.'

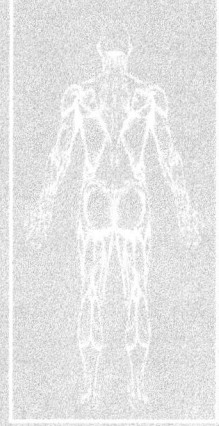

6
Muscle Sections

A s has been established, unilateral resistance training of a prime moving muscle is the foundation of the BMC Training System. The next step, once a muscle has been nominated for exercise, is dividing it into sections (for training purposes).

The theory behind – and the advantage of – dividing a muscle into sections stems from the fact that some muscles may execute more than one function, have more than one head (that is, origin attachment) and subsequent function. As well, they may be made up of different portions that converge into a common tendon and have multi-functions that require varied positions for contraction. One such example is the deltoid or shoulder muscle. It is divided into three portions which converge into a common tendon:

1. *anterior deltoid,* which flexes and inwardly rotates the arm in a sagittal plane

2. *middle deltoid*, which abducts the arm in a coronal plane

3. *posterior deltoid*, which abducts and extends the arm in a transverse plane.

'If you want to know which muscle or muscle aspect
you are contracting, just touch it!'

The BMC Training System divides and isolates a prime moving muscle into four aspects for exercise (by way of example, see Figure 6.1 for the four aspects of a biceps muscle):

1. *superior*, the uppermost fibres of a muscle

2. *inferior*, the lowermost fibres of a muscle

3. *lateral*, the outermost fibres of a muscle

4. *medial*, the innermost fibres of a muscle.

The advantages of exercising a prime moving muscle in aspects are that it:

- caters to the previously mentioned issues relating to muscles

- heightens focus during muscle contraction

- guarantees that a prime moving muscle is contracted through its full range of motion

- ensures optimal development in size, strength and conditioning in a safe and efficient manner

- bypasses the biomechanical deficiencies of some resistance machines

- exposes areas of weakness, most noticeably as uncontrollable shaking and lack of strength during exercise.

Figure 6.1 Aspects of a biceps muscle (a) superior, lateral fibres (b) superior, medial fibres
(c) Inferior, lateral fibres   (d) Inferior, medial fibres

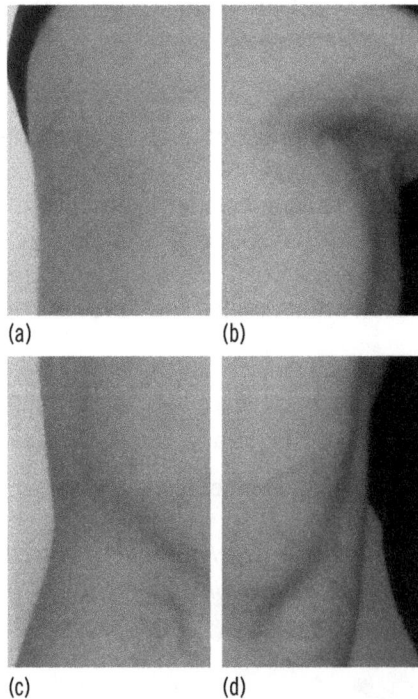

(a)   (b)

(c)   (d)

Mind–muscle Connection: Finding the Aspect

Nominating a prime moving muscle and exercise is one thing; a mind–muscle connection is needed to bring the two together. The mind–muscle connection is a heightened level of awareness, focused on achieving optimal and efficient contraction of a prime moving muscle and its aspects during a resistance exercise.

Closing the eyes, palpating the muscle and executing an abnormal number of sets and repetitions are three ways of connecting or locating an aspect of a muscle. They help to make the mind–muscle connection.

Closing the Eyes

Closing the eyes during an exercise allows better focus on muscle contraction. Safety precautions are imperative to avoid accidents and injuries: first become familiar with surroundings, limit weight used during exercise, and keep the ego in check. Start with a simple movement with the eyes closed, **never** using maximum resistance. Professional supervisors will decide if this strategy is appropriate for those aged under 18, with mental or physical disadvantage, or with no experience in resistance training.

Palpating a Muscle

Palpating a muscle – touching or feeling it – enables accurate fine tuning of a contraction. For safety and accuracy, analysing a muscle contraction by these means should always be carried out when there is no form of resistance. Success with this type of procedure requires a good understanding of muscle anatomy.

(*Note:* In some circumstances, palpating of a muscle is best done with the help of another person.)

Executing an Abnormal Number of Sets

Any uncertainty as to what muscle or aspect is contracting can be easily clarified by executing an abnormal number of sets or repetitions of an exercise to which a prime moving muscle is unaccustomed, creating a state of exhaustion or over-training.

The end result or outcome will be muscle soreness or pain, generally in the following days; this will indicate the exact muscle fibres that have been exercised.

Over time and with experience, the mind–muscle connection can be achieved not only through learning but also through the analysis of shape, function and appropriate position required for a prime moving muscle.

Table 6.1: Reasons for exercising a muscle in aspects.

ACTION	Guarantees the full length of a muscle is contracted, as a muscle may carry out more than one action or function.
INERTIA	Bypasses inertia, allowing continuous contraction without resistance to motion (see Section Three, Chapter 9)
ACCELERATED MOMENTUM	Bypasses inertia, reducing the need for accelerated momentum which, in turn, maximises optimal muscle contraction (see Section Two; see also Section Three, Chapter 10)
INJURY	Reduces the potential for injury to soft tissue and joints by avoiding the use of accelerated momentum.

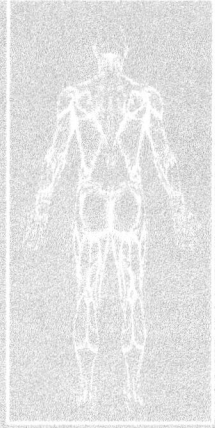

Ideal Position

I t is imperative that any muscle used during a resistance exercise contracts in an unrestricted and natural range of movement. Through ignorance or poor guidance, one can quickly develop the habit of incorrectly, unproductively – even dangerously – positioning body parts during exercise. This may damage muscles, joints and connective tissue without one even realising it.

The ideal position for a prime moving muscle begins with balance. Balance is the act of keeping body parts other than the prime moving muscle motionless from any generated force. Balance creates stability and a solid foundation for executing a strong pull or push contraction during a resistance exercise.

The key to balance and stability during a resistance exercise is alignment of the body and supporting structure. Ideally, alignment occurs when the centre of body mass and the supporting structure correspond; deviation from alignment can affect optimal balance and stability.

Placing the body and prime moving muscle in the correct position for contraction during an exercise ultimately leads to energy efficiency, increased performance, decreased injury potential and optimal muscle development.

'If it does not feel right generally this means that it's not right.
Not feeling right can mean pain, discomfort, general irritation and a lack
of desire to execute or continue with an exercise.'

Elements of Position

To achieve the best possible position during an exercise so that mechanical advantage, balance and safety are attained, the function of a prime moving muscle, synovial joint and resistance equipment must be taken into account. The following elements dictate the optimal position of a prime moving muscle during a resistance exercise:

1. origin/insertion attachment points of a muscle

2. angle in which the muscle fibres run between the attachment points

3. multiple heads or origin attachment point

4. muscle fibres running in different directions, such as the deltoid muscle

5. muscle aspect – upper, lower, outer or inner fibres.

The key element of position, which ultimately dictates directional movement and subsequent position of a prime moving muscle, is the synovial joint. Synovial joints of the human body have different shapes, and different functions that create movement in varied ranges.

The shape or design of a particular piece of resistance equipment (depending on the manufacturing company) – which may have adjustable parts such as the seat, back rest, leg pads, range limiting devices, adjustable pulleys, etc. – will determine in what position a prime moving muscle can be placed or the range of motion executed.

(*Note:* An obvious but very important factor that must be taken into consideration is that people come in various shapes and sizes! This limits the 'one size fits all' scenario in relation to equipment use.)

Body Parts and Position

Irrespective of what prime moving muscle is nominated, there are three areas of the body that are pivotal to executing resistance exercises: the hands, feet and pelvis.

Without them it would be impossible to create a position to optimally contract the prime moving muscle (or aspects); to grasp equipment; or to stand, lie, sit or balance during an exercise.

(*Note:* Hand, foot, limb or body part position during exercises outlined in Section Four are specific to muscle and/or muscle aspects, catering for optimal contraction in an efficient and safe manner.)

Hands

In the BMC Training System, the hands have simultaneous but separate roles: one (the working hand) is used to execute the exercise while the other supports and balances the body. Placing the hand in a position for exercise requires movement of either the elbow or shoulder joints; the specific hand position depends on the prime moving muscle (or aspect) nominated for contraction.

There are six hand positions (Figure 7.1):

a. prone, palm down

b. semi-prone, palm down at a 45° angle

c. neutral (thumb up); in between prone and supine

d. semi-supine, palm up at a 45° angle

e. supine, palm up

f. neutral (thumb down); in between prone and supine.

Figure 7.1 Hand positions (a) prone (b) semi-prone (c) neutral (thumb up) (d) semi-supine (e) supine (f) neutral (thumb down)

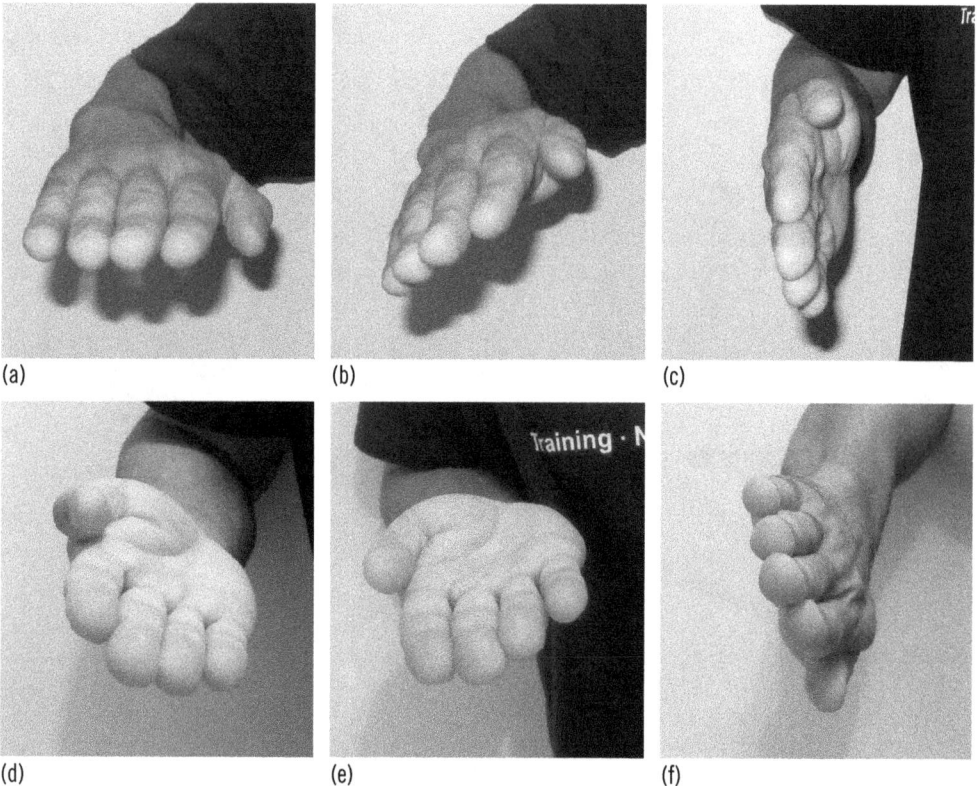

Feet

Much like the hands, the feet have simultaneous but separate roles: one (the working foot) is used to execute the exercise while the other supports and balances the body.

Placing the foot in a position for exercise requires movement of either the ankle or hip joints; the specific foot position depends on the prime moving muscle (or aspect) nominated for contraction.

There are five main foot positions (Figure 7.2)

a. invert, toes pointing inward
b. neutral, toes pointing straight ahead
c. evert, toes pointing outward
d. dorsiflexion, toes pointing upward
e. plantar flexion, toes pointing downward.

Figure 7.2 Foot positions (a) invert (b) neutral (c) evert (d) dorsiflexion (e) plantar flexion

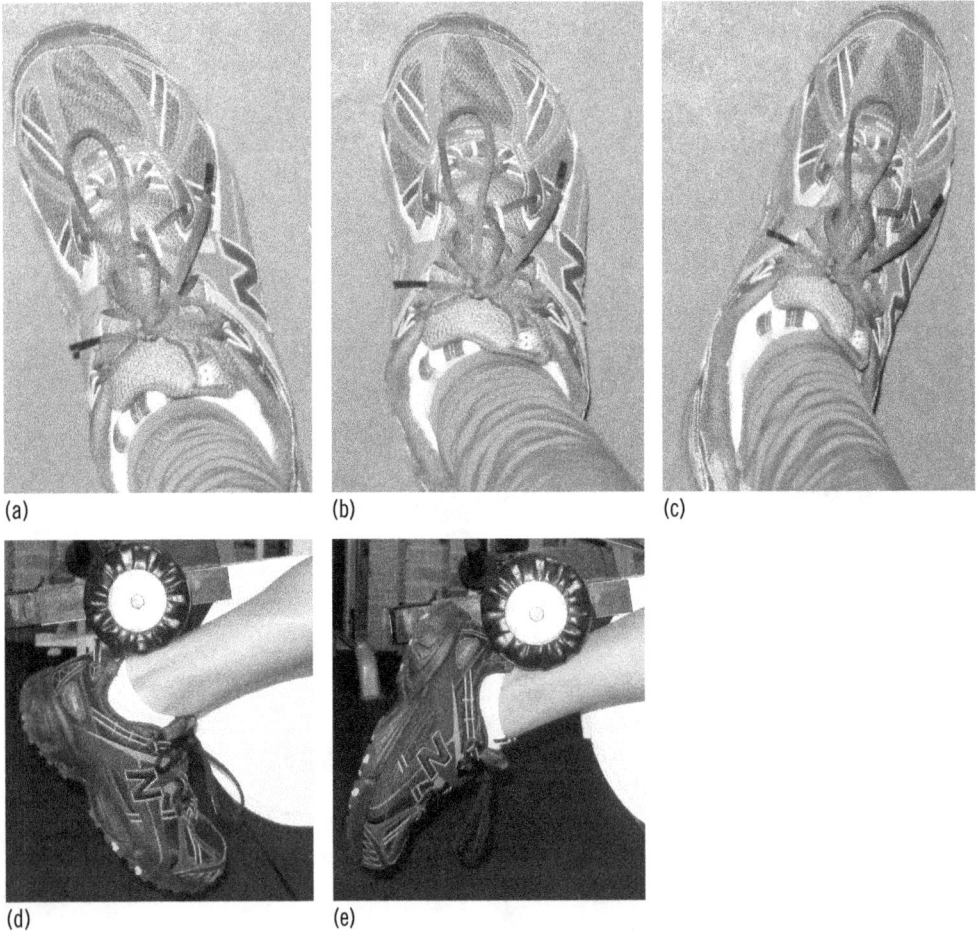

(a)　　　　　　　　　(b)　　　　　　　　　(c)

(d)　　　　　　　　　(e)

Pelvis

The pelvis is an area of great importance as it allows rotational movement of the upper and lower body, catering for a unilateral position.

When a leg is brought forward (Figure 7.3(b)), the pelvis rotates, moving that particular side into an anterior position and the opposite side into a posterior position.

The role of the pelvis differs from that of the hands and feet in most instances as it functions purely as a support for the body.

Exercise Positions

There are three positions (and associated variations) that the BMC Training System adopts for its resistance exercises: standing, seated and lying.

The position assumed will depend on the muscle, exercise and equipment involved. Ultimately, the goal of each exercise position is to achieve maximum balance and leverage so that a safe and optimal muscle contraction is ensured.

Standing Position

There are two standing positions that can be assumed during resistance exercise: bilateral or unilateral (Figure 7.3).

a. The bilateral stance: a position in which the left and right leg are aligned with each other; generally occurs at either a shoulder- or hip-width stance. This particular stance caters for bilateral exercises either as a support mechanism or as a means of working a muscle, evenly distributing the resistance weight on either side of the body.

b. The unilateral stance: a position in which the left leg is placed forward and the right leg placed backward (or vice versa) in a diagonal fashion with feet facing forward is the fundamental stance of the BMC Training System; it caters specifically for unilateral exercise. **(When an exercise is carried out with the right arm, place the left foot forward and the right foot backward – and vice versa when exercising with the other arm.)**

(*Note:* Executing a unilateral exercise in a bilateral stance is both unproductive and unsafe; it creates poor balance and leverage and ultimately places unnecessary pressure on the lower back through uneven weight distribution.)

Figure 7.3 (a) Bilateral stance (b) Unilateral stance, with left pelvic girdle forward and right backward

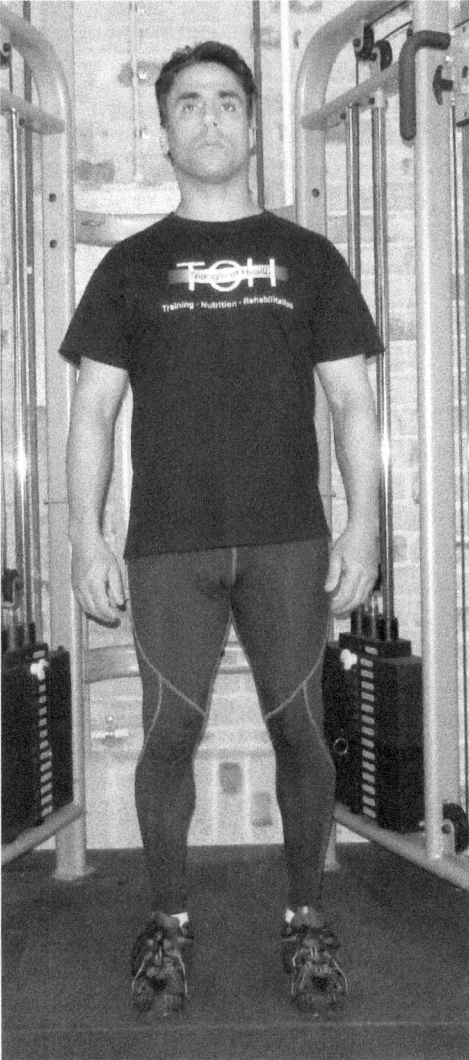 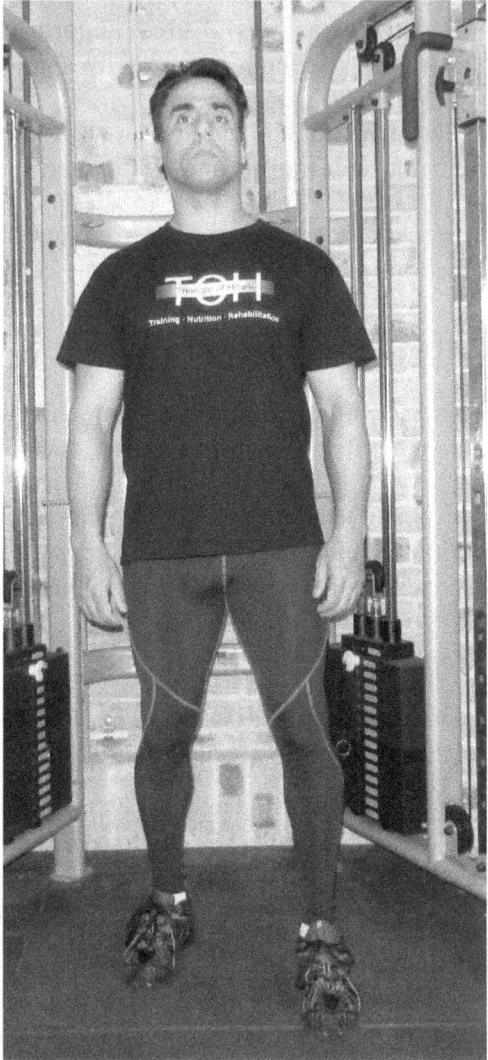

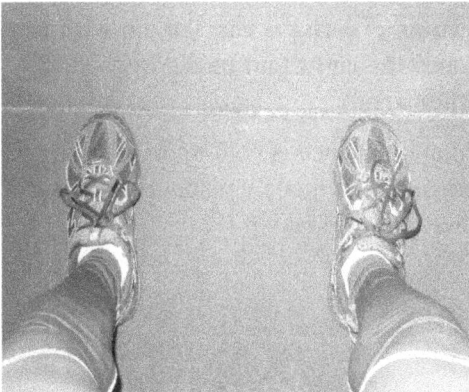 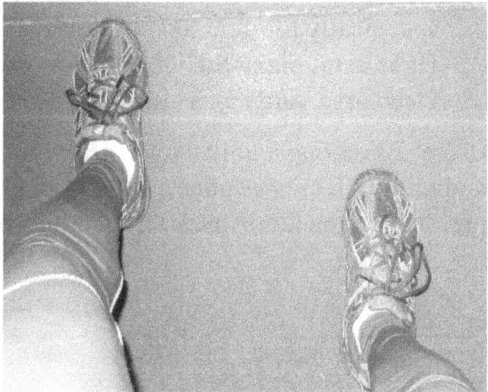

(a)   (b)

Seated Position

The seated positions mimic those of the standing positions: a bilateral stance is a square seated position (Figure 7.4(a)), with the feet aligned at either a hip or shoulder width.

The other seated position has half the pelvis rotating forward (Figure 7.4(b)) and the other backward, much like the unilateral stance standing position.

Figure 7.4 Seated positions (a) square seated position (b) rotated seated position

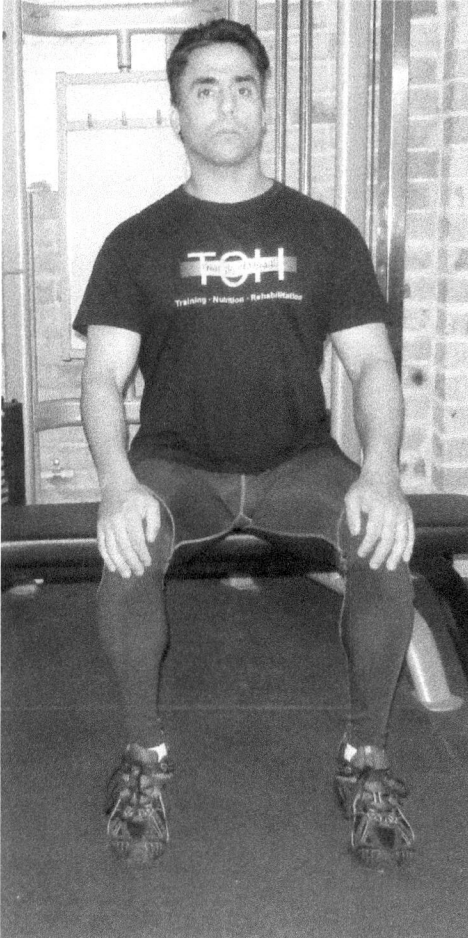 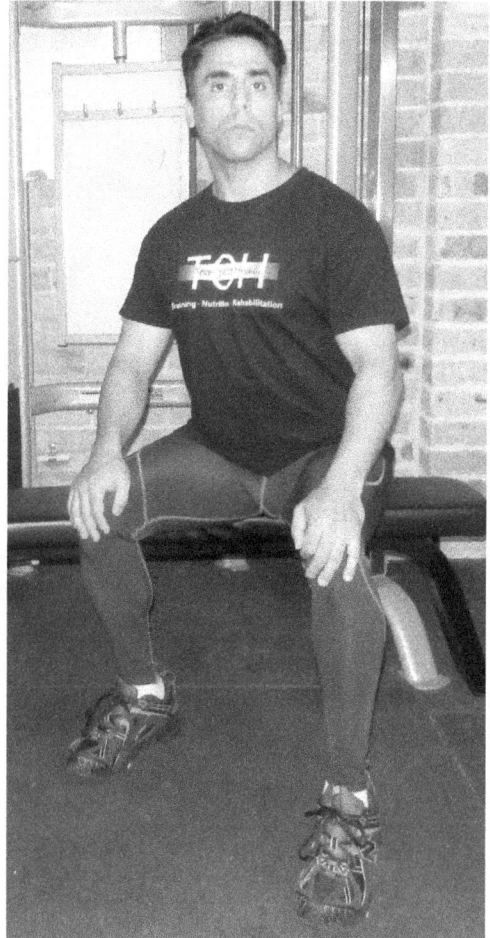

(a)   (b)

Lying Position

There are three lying positions:

a.   prone, lying on the front of the body facing in a downward direction

b.   supine, lying on the back of the body facing in a upward direction

c.   neutral, lying on the side of the body (see Figure 7.5).

Figure 7.5 Lying positions (a) prone (b) supine (c) neutral

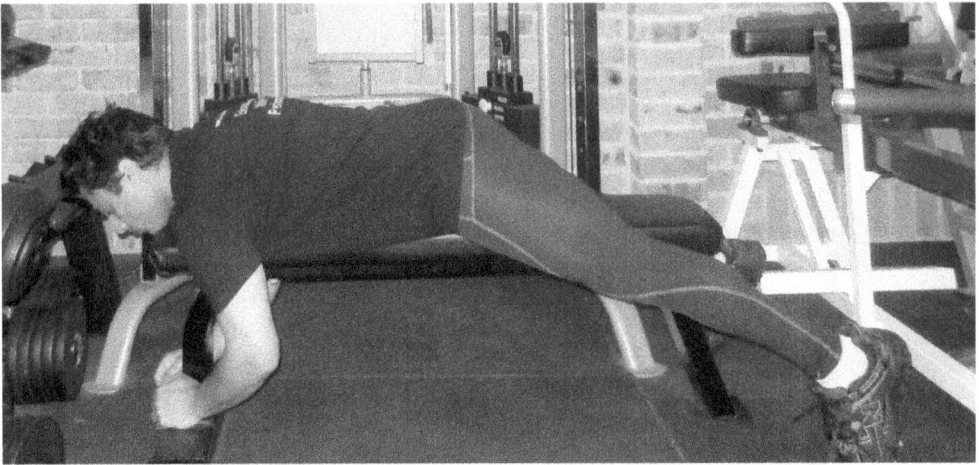

(a)

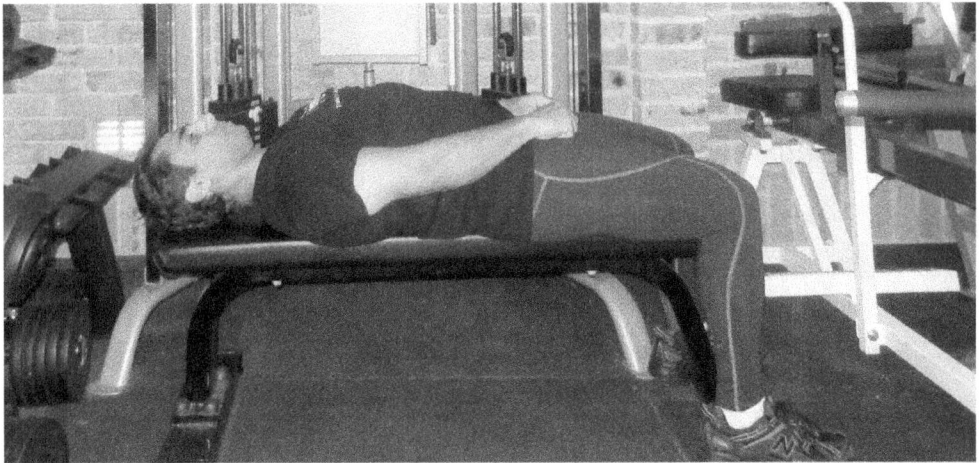

(b)

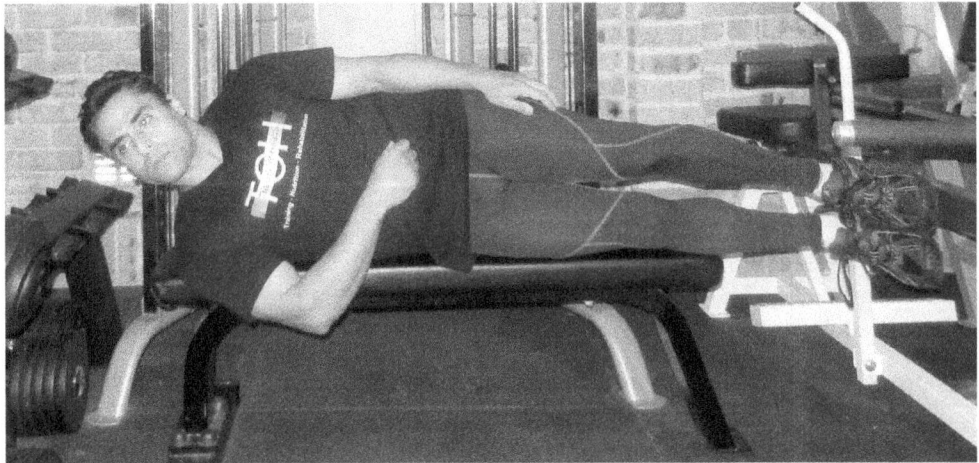

(c)

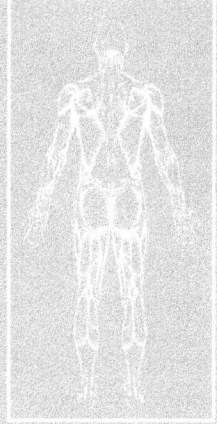

8
Movement Pattern

T he objective of any resistance exercise should be to develop muscles in a safe and efficient manner. This is best achieved by contracting a prime moving muscle through a natural, uninhibited path known as the movement pattern The BMC Training System recognises that the fundamental aspect of a movement pattern is the natural action of a prime moving muscle and related joint(s). Other components, such as position, direction and motion, are, however, also very important.

Habitual, inappropriate movement patterns over time are a recipe for acute or chronic injury. Symptoms of an abnormal movement pattern, short or long term, are muscle tightness, muscle strain and movement restriction, joint inflammation and pain.

'The ideal movement pattern is one in which the contracting prime moving muscle, corresponding joint(s) and exercise equipment or apparatus move in a natural, uninhibited path that is comfortable, smooth and pain free to execute.'

Determining how to execute a movement pattern starts by nominating a prime moving muscle and its specific aspect. Choosing the aspect will dictate the appropriate implementation of key movement pattern components such as position, direction and motion during resistance exercise.

Position

The position component of a movement pattern relates to the angle in which a prime moving muscle, joint, limb – and body as a whole – are placed.

Ultimately, it is the synovial joints that allow movement to occur and that dictate the position of limbs or body parts for the start of an exercise.

In some instances, a specific joint function can be carried out by multiple muscles, necessitating varied limb, hand or feet positions. One such example is flexing or bending of the lower arm at the elbow joint which can be carried out by the biceps, brachialis and brachioradialis muscles (Figure 8.1) through varied shoulder, elbow and hand positions.

Figure 8.1 Elbow joint flexors   (a) biceps (hand supine) (b) brachialis (hand semi-prone)
(c) brachioradialis (hand neutral)

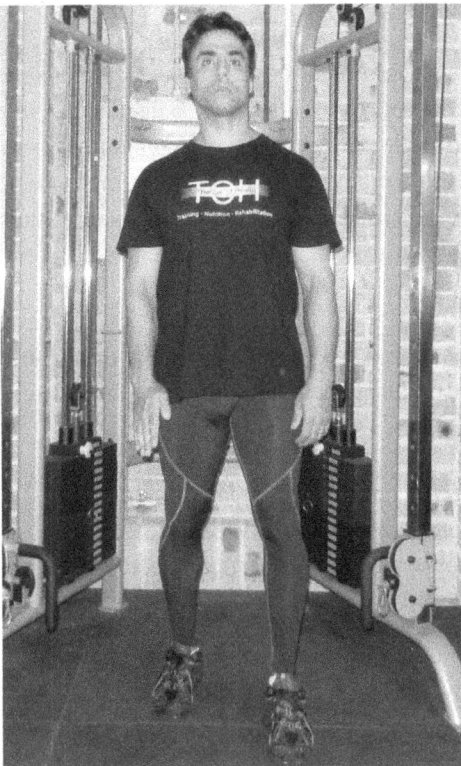

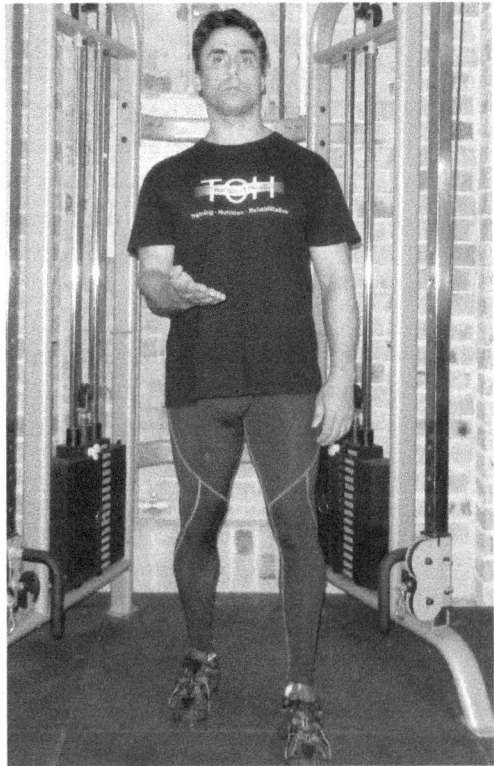

(a)

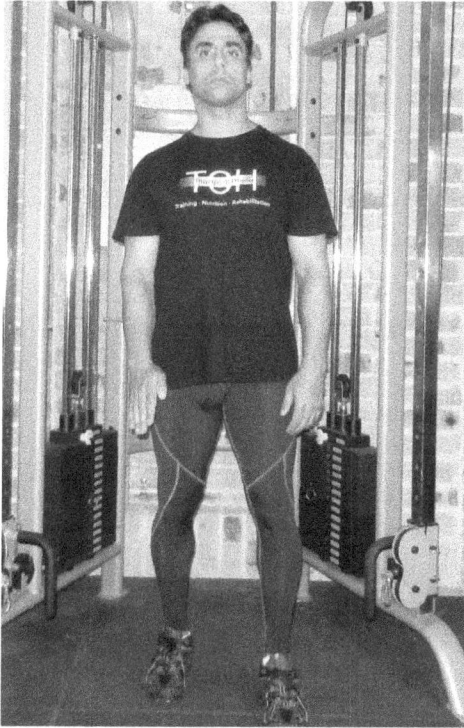
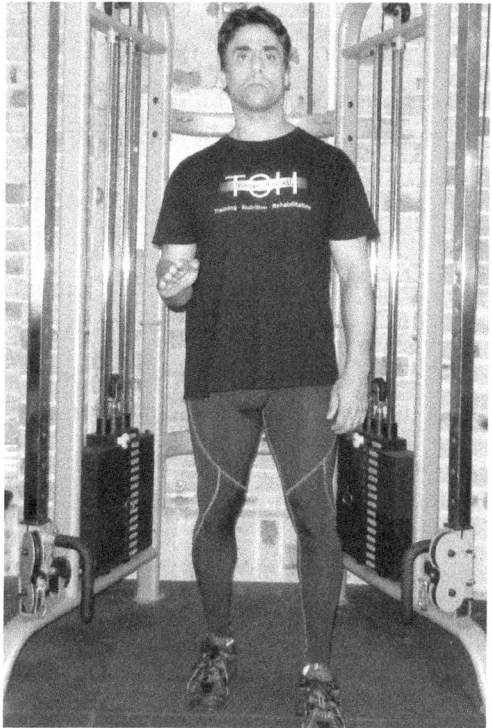

(b)

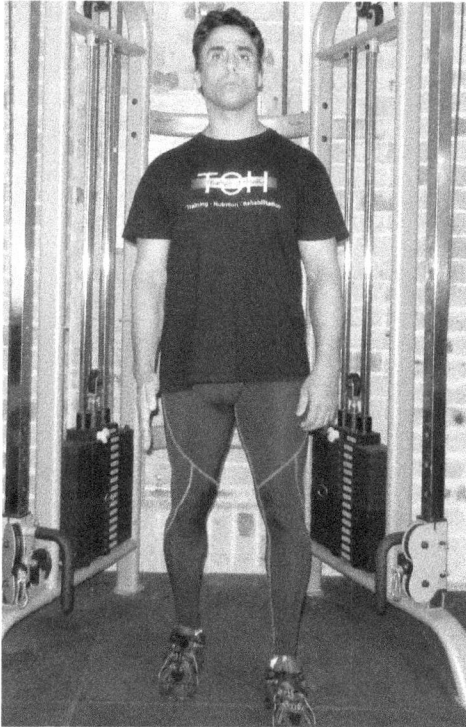
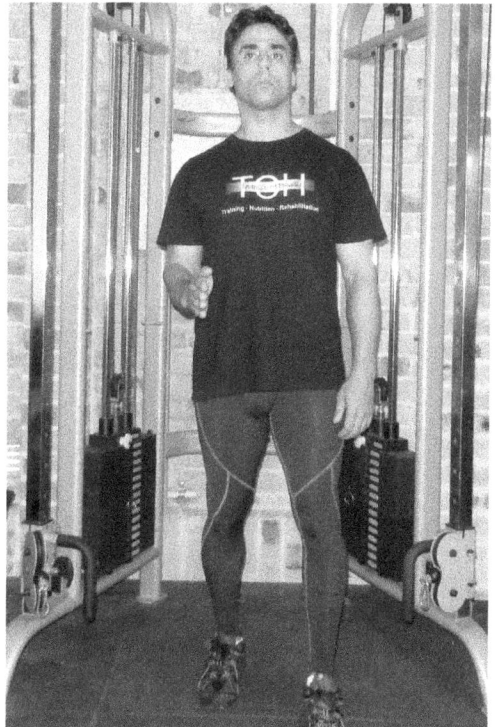

(c)

Direction

The direction component of a movement pattern refers to the plane in which a prime moving muscle and its associated structures move.

Viewed as a three-dimensional structure, the human body is bisected by imaginary lines creating the sagittal, coronal and transverse planes (Figure 8.2).

- The sagittal plane is the direction in which a vertical line passes through the body from front to back or vice versa, dividing it into equal left and right sides.

- The coronal plane is the direction in which a vertical line passes through the body from a side to side position, dividing it into equal front and back sides.

- The transverse plane is the direction in which a horizontal line passes through the body, from front to back or side to side, dividing it into equal top and bottom halves.

All three planes meet at the centre of the body at right angles to each other; this meeting point is the centre of body mass. Irrespective of whether a contracting muscle creates movement of a limb, body part or resistance apparatus in a forward, backward, outward, inward, or up or down manner, the directional path will always be in one or more of the above-mentioned planes.

Figure 8.2 Planes of the body and exercise movement (a) sagittal (b) coronal (c) transverse

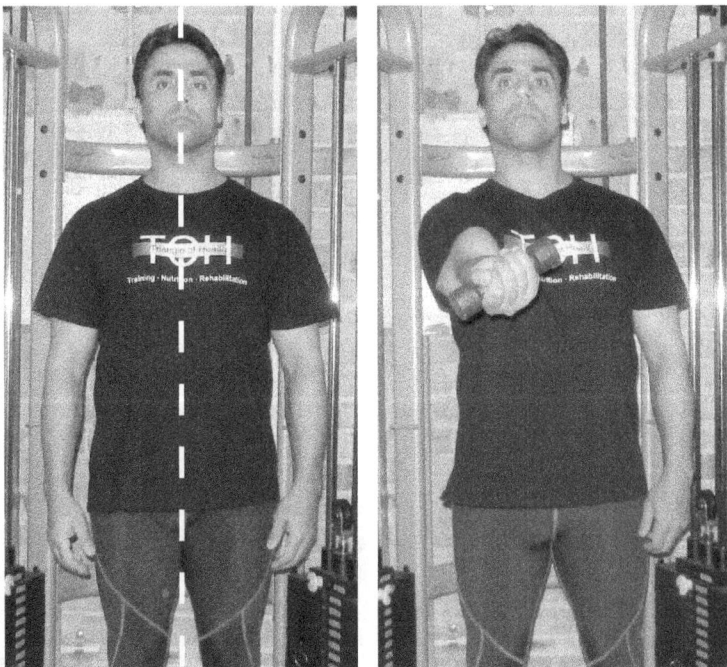

(a)

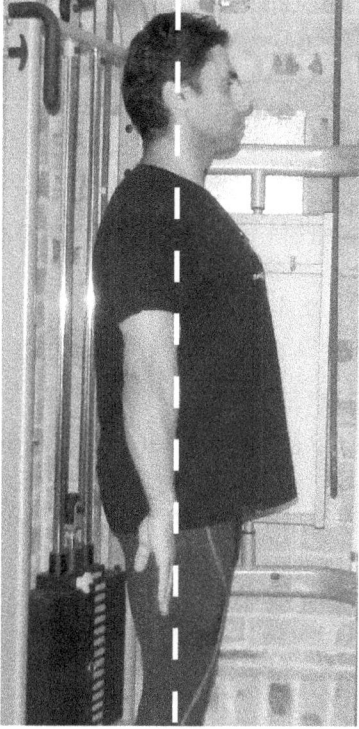
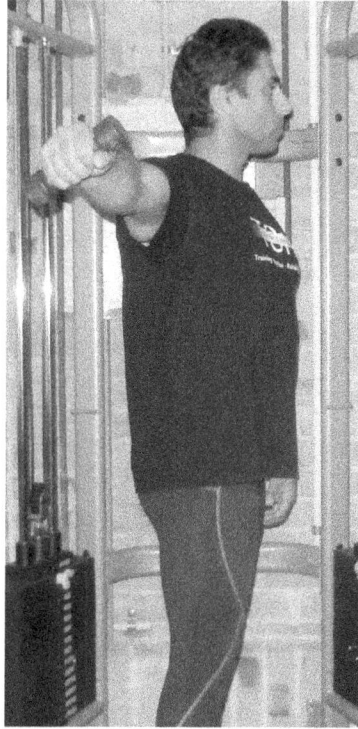

(b)

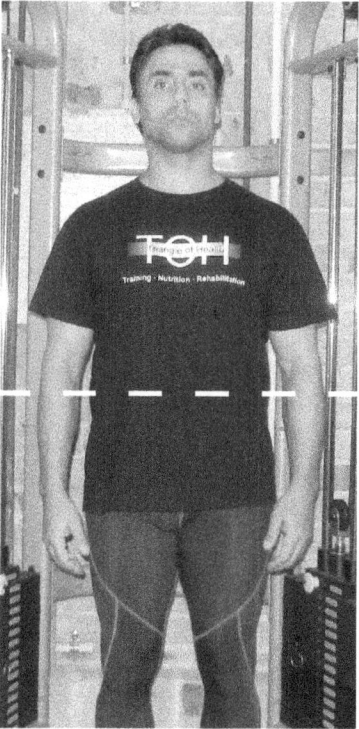
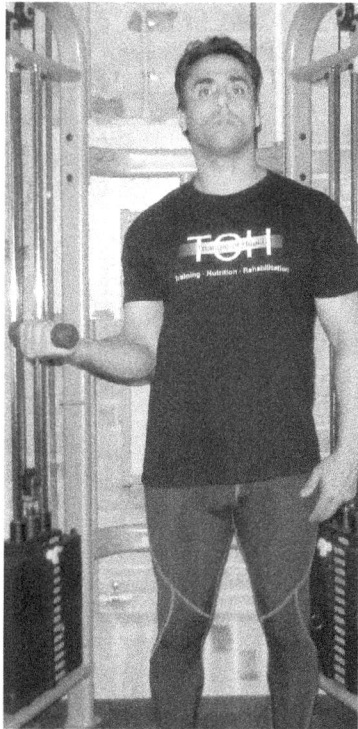

(c)

Motion

The BMC Training System deems that a prime moving muscle should be contracted through a full range of motion – but not in the long-established manner to which most are accustomed.

Traditional full range of motion – the act of movement from beginning to end, created in a single muscle contraction – is commonly known in resistance training as a repetition. A repetition can be created in different lines, different directions and for varying degrees of length, depending on the exercise and piece of resistance equipment used.

The word 'line' tends to conjure up thoughts of a path that is linear (or straight) in direction (Figure 8.3), but such a path is contrary to the curved line that limbs and body parts naturally create. Dictated by shape, structure and attachment point, muscles, bones and connective tissue collectively create a curvilinear (or curved line) of motion (Figure 8.4).

Contraction of a muscle and its associated body parts thus occurs in a convex-shaped (outward) curve or arc line; movement created is in either a medial or lateral direction to the body.

Resistance equipment such as dumbbells and adjustable cable-pulley machines perfectly cater for such movement, with the degree of curve during movement depending on the:

- synovial joint (type)
- muscle function
- exercise position
- range of motion
- equipment used.

(*Note:* Movement created during an exercise using a traditional full-range-of-motion muscle contraction with equipment that functions in a linear line (Figure 8.3) defies natural biomechanics; over time, this will cause structural problems and injuries.)

Figure 8.3 Leg press carriage – movement in a linear line

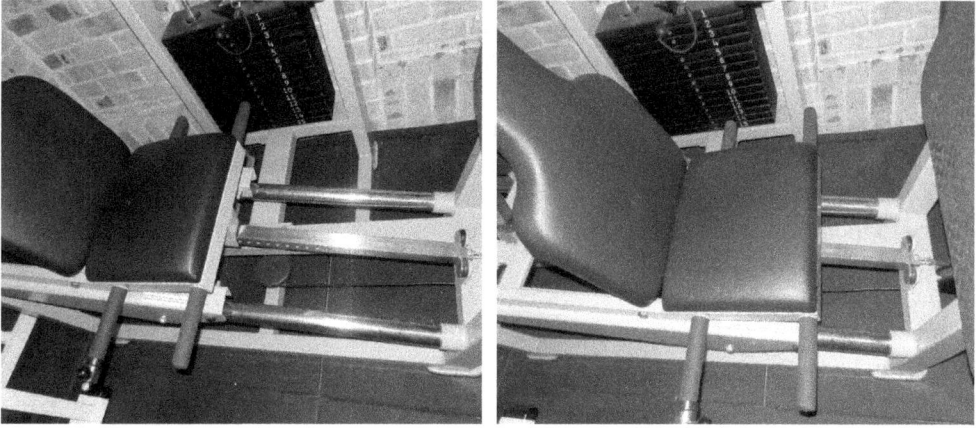

Figure 8.4 Curvilinear path of a dumbbell curl

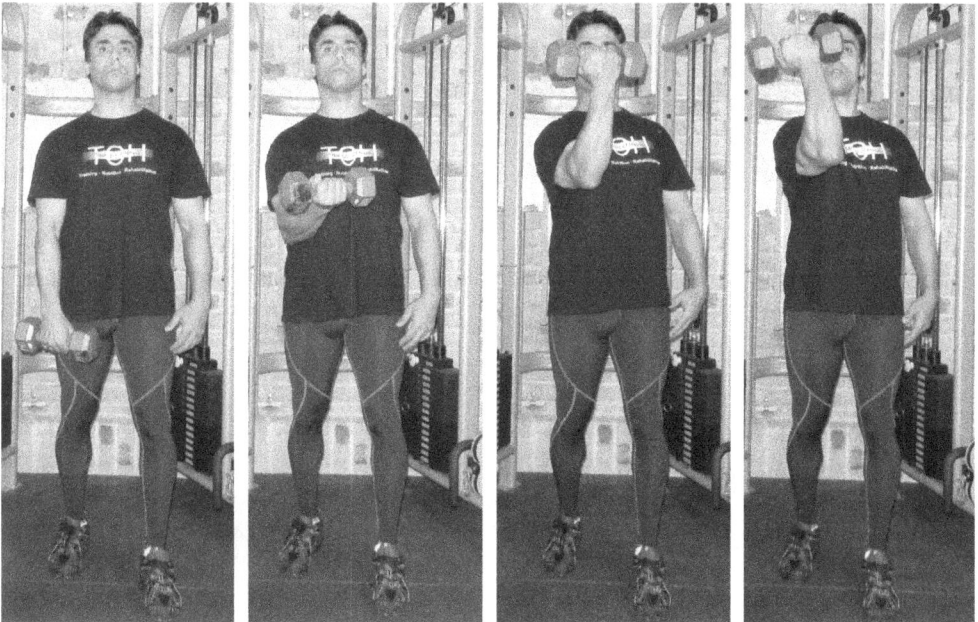

Range of Motion

Range of motion (ROM) is the distance travelled when a muscle contracts, creating movement of a limb or body part via a joint.

The ideal ROM for muscle development and proper function is a debate that has been raging for many years among resistance training enthusiasts.

To try to identify the ideal ROM in resistance training, the first question that must be addressed is: What is normal?

A muscle attaches at two points onto a skeletal structure: via the origin (the fixed point) and insertion (the moving point), with at least one point attaching across a joint. When a muscle contracts, it moves between the two points, moving the relevant structures of attachment toward each other. It is the coming together of the structures that determines the most appropriate ROM.

When structures come together, it is important that the meeting is subtle, ceasing at the first point of contact or before, but not beyond. Anything past the point of contact creates a hyper-movement (Figure 8.5(b)) of the associated joint, which in the short or long term can lead to possible damage to muscles, connective tissue or bone structures. A natural, safe and productive ROM can be characterised by a couple of degrees of space between two articulating bones.

Figure 8.5 (a) Normal full extension of lower arm at elbow joint (b) Hyper-extension of lower arm at elbow joint

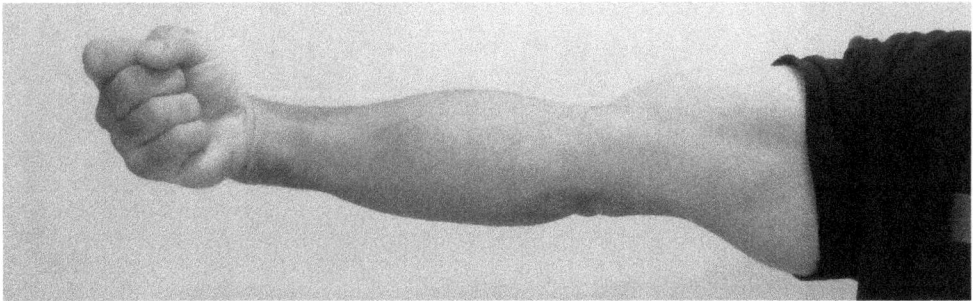

(a)

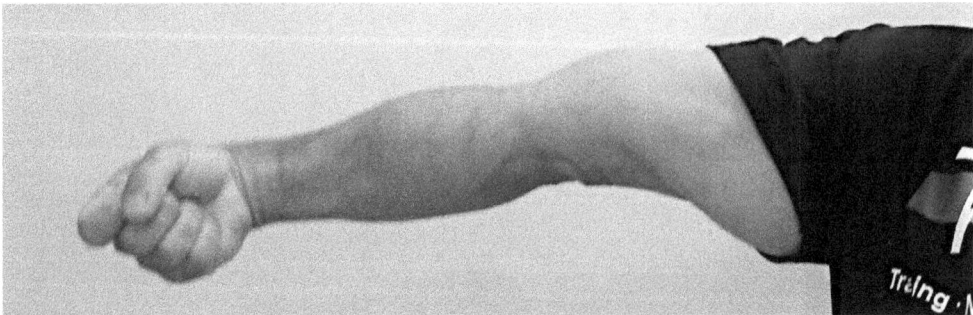

(b)

A muscle contraction's ROM during resistance exercise can be executed in a full or partial manner.

The concept of a full ROM can be misleading, and confusing, a problem stemming from a perception of necessary movement. The confusion arises because some consider that a full ROM is not complete until the associated limb (or body part structure) of a contracting prime moving muscle has completed the full distance it is capable of moving.

Focus on full ROM should primarily be on the prime moving muscle ceasing at peak contraction (Figure 8.6), with its associated structures doing so as well.

The flaws of a traditional full ROM muscle contraction are:

- the temptation for accelerated momentum which, in turn, increases risk of injury and decreases proper muscle development
- mechanical disadvantage
- the increased likelihood of inertia
- the tendency for a muscle to fatigue faster.

Short ROM is defined as a partial muscle contraction with the following advantages:

- decreased need for accelerated momentum which, in turn, decreases the risk of injury and allows complete muscle development
- greater mechanical advantage
- avoidance of inertia
- muscle fatigue resistance
- increased focus on muscle aspect.

Figure 8.6 (a) Peak contraction of biceps muscle (b) Hyper-flexion: abnormal contraction of biceps muscle

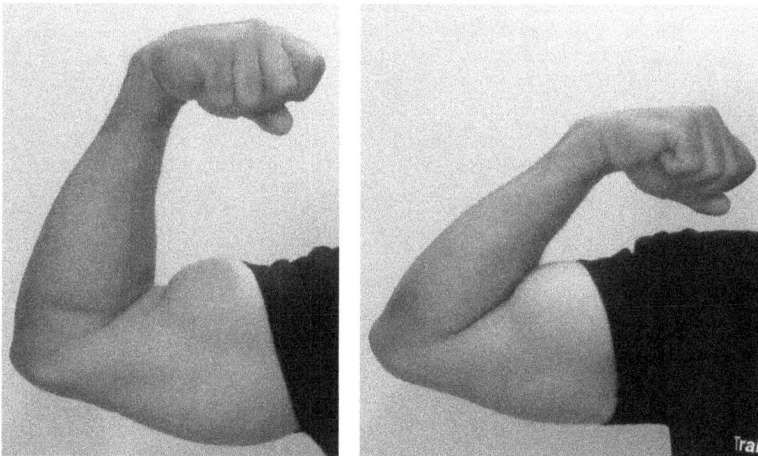

(a) (b)

Table 8.1: Important considerations that can increase or limit the ROM of a muscle, joint, limb or other body part.

MUSCLE	JOINT	LIMB
Aspect or Section: The deltoid muscle is an example where the middle portion allows a greater range of arm movement at the shoulder joint than the anterior or posterior portion of the muscle.	**Type:** The synovial joint type will affect ROM. The shoulder joint, an example of a ball and socket joint, caters to a large and varied ROM, while a hinge joint like the knee is restrictive in comparison.	**Position:** Using a limb to execute a resistance exercise in a straight or bent manner can increase or decrease ROM.
Function: The biceps muscle bending the lower arm at the elbow joint travels a greater distance than the rhomboid muscle adducting the scapula.	**Connective Structure:** Synovial joint soft tissue structures, such as joint capsules and ligaments, dictate not only the ROM but also directional movement. An example is the shoulder joint: the joint capsule is fixed loosely at the bottom of the humeral head of the upper arm bone (allowing greater range of motion during abduction of the arm); at the top, it is fixed tightly, restricting flexion of the arm across the body. Ligaments of the shoulder are positioned in such a way that allow greater internal rotation and restrict external rotation.	
Structure: Muscles made up of a long muscle belly and short tendons decrease ROM, while those with a short muscle belly and long tendons increase ROM. Greater muscle belly girth also affects ROM, decreasing where two structural points meet.		
Injury: This will shorten muscle fibres, consequently affecting normal ROM.		

Segment Motion

The ideal ROM is one that removes the disadvantages of a traditional full ROM and employs the advantages of a short ROM, which subsequently develops a muscle through the full length of its fibres.

To achieve this, the BMC Training System uses a muscle contraction referred to as segment motion. Segment motion (Figure 8.7) is the complete contraction of a prime moving muscle, with the distance covered in two separate segments or parts.

Controlling the ROM in segments allows a muscle to contract under constant tension, maintaining a firmness better known as peak contraction, which leads to a better conditioned muscle.

Figure 8.7 Executing a dumbbell curl in two segments, avoiding inertia and accelerated momentum

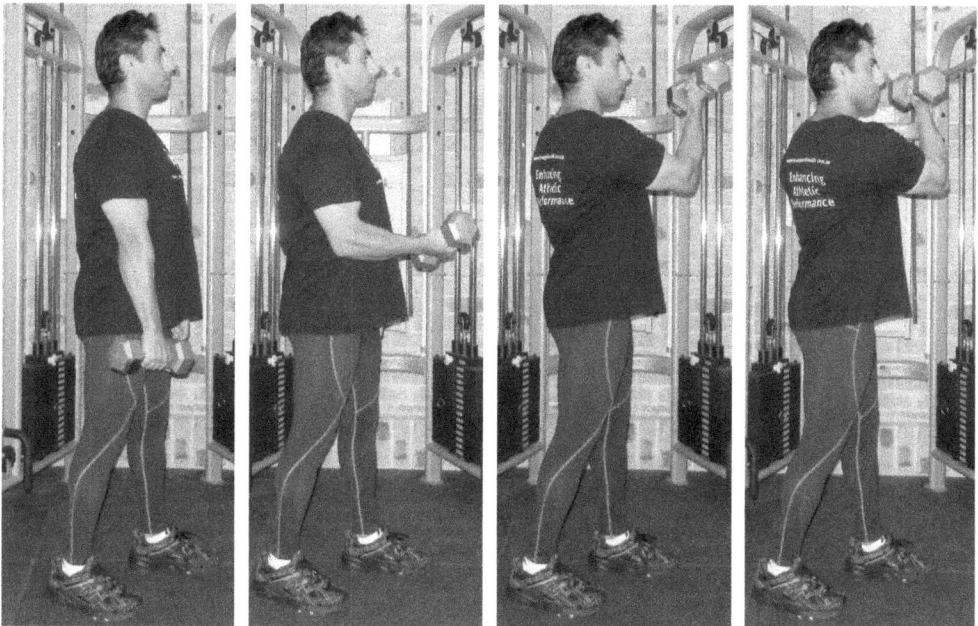

(a) lower start   (b) lower finish   (c) upper start   (d) upper finish

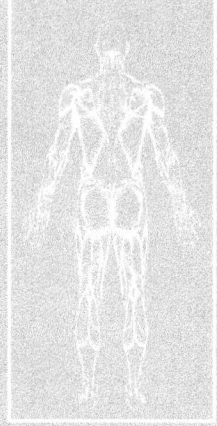

9
Inertia

Another issue that can interfere with a muscle's completing a smooth, uninhibited full ROM contraction is inertia. Inertia is the resistance point of motion during an exercise, commonly referred to in bodybuilding circles as the 'sticking point' – the point at which movement momentarily or completely ceases during a full ROM muscle contraction due to a weight or load. The interference that inertia creates stems from either one or a combination of the following: the weight used during exercise, gravity, and/or muscle fatigue.

Weight raised or lowered during an exercise is done so against the force of gravity. In conjunction with gravity, inertia is influenced by speed, weight, muscle strength and position. Contracting a muscle slowly, coupled with a heavy weight and/or decreased muscle strength, increases the likelihood of inertia, as does positioning resistance away from the centre of body mass, decreasing mechanical leverage. Inertia can sabotage the full benefits resistance training has to offer and is the main reason why people instinctively use accelerated momentum to continue to finish a muscle contraction.

'The obvious is not always apparent.'

Point of Inertia

Using accelerated momentum to overcome inertia is problematic, as it removes the emphasis on the efficient and complete contraction of a prime moving muscle; this affects development and increases the risk of injury. Inertia is the main reason why segment motion muscle contraction is an integral part of the BMC Training System — contracting a prime moving muscle in segments endeavours to avoid what is referred to as point of inertia (POI) (Figure 9.1).

The benefits of avoiding POI are that it:

- allows optimal contraction of a prime moving muscle, without the temptation for accelerated momentum

- allows better isolation of – and constant tension to be placed upon – the prime moving muscle, as well as better control of resistance weight.

- decreases the fatigue factor, allowing a prime moving muscle to go beyond its normal capabilities

- decreases the risk of injury

- increases mechanical leverage and energy efficiency.

Figure 9.1 POI, also known as the 'sticking point'

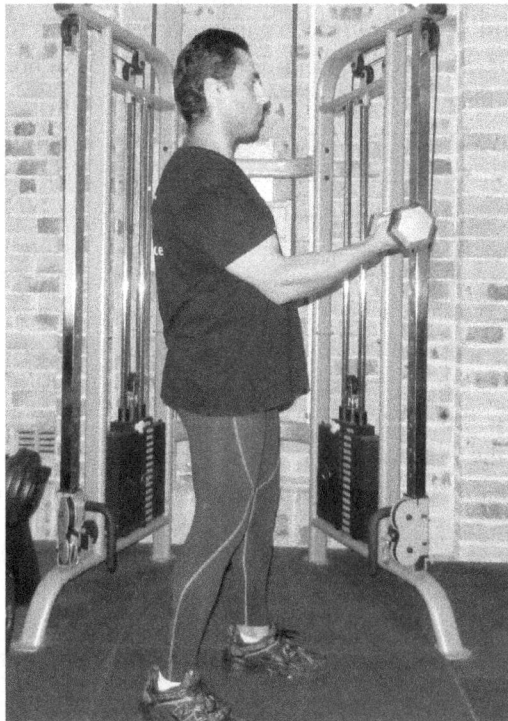

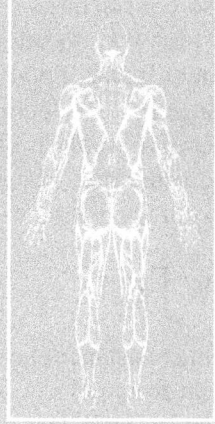

10
How Fast? How Much?
How Hard?

How? This simple word starts some important questions, listed below, about the BMC Training System.

How fast? – relates to the speed of a muscle contraction and the tempo with which a resistance weight should move.

How much? – relates to the amount of weight, work rate or volume of exercise (in the form of sets and repetitions and the rest period between exercises and sets) used by a prime moving muscle.

How hard? – relates to the effort or intensity carried out during an exercise.

Answers to these three questions will vary for each individual in the light of a range of variables: sleep, illness, chemical enhancement (legal and illegal), emotional stress, food consumption and nutritional value, water consumption, alcohol consumption, cigarette habits, air pollution and others. One or a combination of any of these variables can affect energy levels and enthusiasm on a daily basis, altering how an individual will feel, function and appear.

'Can you afford to ignore the truth?'

These considerations thus make these simple questions more difficult to answer. The best way to attempt to do so is to follow your instincts and use logic and common sense. Following your instincts means making decisions based on natural feelings (or 'gut feelings') rather than on specific information or reasoning. This is imperative, as each person's body is constantly changing, and these changes need to be addressed. Listening to how one's body feels and functions during any given workout is paramount for safety and progress.

How Fast?

During resistance exercise, a prime moving muscle will contract, moving a nominated weight from point A to point B. The speed with which a weight moves between the two points will depend on the type of muscle contraction.

The isotonic muscle contraction is made up of two separate contractions, concentric and eccentric. These are the main muscle contractions used in resistance training.

- The concentric contraction, also known as the positive repetition, is the phase in which muscle fibres shorten during movement of a weight in a moderately quick fashion.

- In contrast, the eccentric contraction, also known as the negative repetition, is the phase in which muscle fibres lengthen during movement of a weight in a moderately slow fashion.

Irrespective of which sort of contraction it is, both must be carried out in a smooth and controlled manner. A repetition can be executed in a slow, fast or ballistic manner with speed from start to finish gauged by time.

- The speed of a slow repetition can vary from 5 to 10 seconds, ensuring control and complete contraction of the prime moving muscle. The problem with executing a slow repetition is the necessary weight reduction of resistance so that inertia can be avoided; this subsequently eliminates the ability for a muscle to work or exercise to its full potential.

- The speed of a fast repetition executed between 1 and 2 seconds (in an attempt to bypass inertia) offers less control of a resistance weight by the prime moving muscle, leading to poor or incomplete muscle contraction; this affects development and increases the potential for injury.

- A ballistic repetition, one that is explosive and created through accelerated momentum, is generally carried out in less than 1 second. This type of repetition fails to focus on the contraction of a prime moving muscle, while, at the same time, it increases the risk of damage to muscles, connective tissue and joints, especially if underlying structural problems are undetected.

The speed of a repetition during an exercise will be influenced by variables such as resistance weight and strength, and conditioning or injury to a prime moving muscle.

Weight of Resistance

The weight of resistance during an exercise will dictate the speed with which a prime moving muscle contracts. Ideally, lifting a light weight should be carried out in a slow, controlled manner, whereas a heavy weight will require a faster speed for efficient movement.

Strength and Conditioning or Injury

A lack of strength and conditioning, or inhibited nerve function, will affect the contraction speed of a muscle.

Another problematic issue associated with repetition speed that must be avoided is accelerated momentum. This has already been stressed. Accelerated momentum, as explained earlier, is the act of moving a weight in a rapid, swinging, uncontrolled manner by the prime moving muscle with the recruited help of other muscles (Figure 10.1).

Accelerated momentum occurs when a prime moving muscle becomes incapable of moving a weight through a reasonable, controlled speed of contraction – a compensatory and instinctive reaction caused generally by either too much weight, muscle fatigue, imbalance or ego or a combination of all four.

The end result of accelerated momentum is a decreased emphasis on the muscle contraction, which subsequently affects the development of a muscle's size, strength and conditioning. This reduces musculoskeletal structural stability.

Continuous Motion Repetition

In conjunction with segment motion, the BMC Training System employs a fast, controlled contraction known as the continuous motion repetition.

Carried out between two short points with a smooth, controlled, rhythmic speed of approximately 1 second, the continuous motion repetition ensures that inertia and hyper-movement of joints are avoided, while providing minimal rest. This subsequently increases muscle conditioning.

Figure 10.1 Accelerated momentum

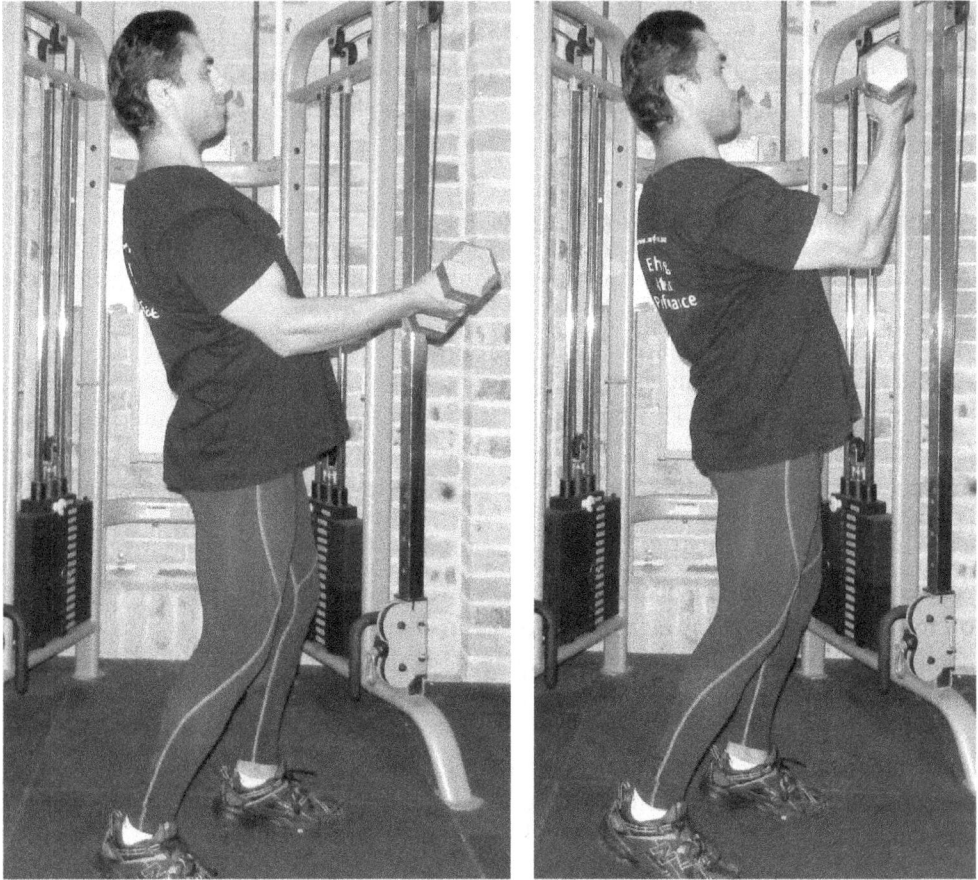

Table 10.1: Contraction speed.

TYPE OF CONTRACTION	SPEED/TIME (SEC)
Concentric	2–3
Eccentric	3–4
Isometric	< 1/10
Fast	1–2
Slow	5–10
Ballistic	< 1

How Much? – Work, Weight, Rest

The question of *How much?* relates to three different areas: volume of work in the form of repetitions and sets, working weight for the prime moving muscle, and the amount of rest required between sets and exercises.

Volume of Work

The volume of work is the nominated number of repetitions and sets carried out for a particular prime moving muscle and exercise. Just as a single muscle contraction is referred to as a repetition (or rep, more commonly), multiple muscle contractions are repetitions or reps.

Repetitions

Repetitions are used to develop size, power, strength, endurance and conditioning of a muscle. They also function as a reference point for gauging muscle strength for a particular weight and exercise.

The number or range of repetitions executed will be dictated by the desired results an individual wishes to achieve with resistance training. Body composition and desired results differ from person to person, making a generic, exact or 'magic number' of repetitions impossible to endorse.

Sets

A set is a predetermined or instinctive number of repetitions executed at one time for a given exercise, with the last repetition signalling the completion of a set. More than one set of an exercise is referred to as sets.

There are various schools of thought about repetition range and the number of sets that one should execute during a workout for a particular muscle and exercise.

Some espouse a 'low number of sets, high-intensity training' philosophy, exercising a muscle in a very hard or intense manner with the sole purpose of exhausting it in a minimal number of sets. Minimal numbers of sets can be problematic, though, as maximum effort in a shorter period of time increases the risk of injury, due to a lack of incremental preparation of the prime moving muscle. Training this way can also cause mental or physical fatigue both in the short and longer term.

Others endorse a 'high volume of sets, moderate intensity training' philosophy, claiming it to be a more efficient, productive and safe way of achieving results.

BMC Training System: Repetitions and Sets

Repetitions and sets in the BMC Training System are unique – quite different from those for traditional bilateral resistance training. This is because the division of a prime moving muscle into upper, lower, outer and inner aspects necessitates multiple segment motion points in moving from point A to B (Figure 10.2). This calculated approach is designed to facilitate maximum muscle development, exercise efficiency and safety.

Exercising a muscle in this manner involves an increased number of sets and repetitions over what a person would normally carry out in bilateral resistance training.

There are two options to pursue for reps and sets when exercising a prime moving muscle in a unilateral fashion: bilateral and unilateral sequence.

- *Bilateral sequence:* A prime moving muscle executes nominated contractions of an aspect, moving from point A to B on one side of the body (starting left or right) without any rest reciprocated on the other side; this concludes a set.

- *Unilateral sequence:* All nominated reps and sets are executed consecutively on one side of the body, then reciprocated on the other. The unilateral sequence is a viable option of increasing training intensity without increasing sets, reps or weight.

Ultimately, the key to achieving desired results is individualised experimentation through trial and error of different repetition ranges and sets.

Table 10.2: Important considerations that affect volume of work.

CONSIDERATION	COMMENT
MUSCLE	• The size and shape of a prime moving muscle will affect the number of sets and reps executed.
	• Bigger muscles generally require more work than smaller muscles, but this also depends on genetics. Some people have muscles that are more responsive, and this needs to be addressed. For example, generally, the quadriceps need more volume of work than the biceps, but genetics may see someone achieve quick results for low volumes for quadriceps, and need more for biceps.
	• A muscle's shape may necessitate multiple exercises for complete development (e.g. the deltoid muscle, made up of three portions: anterior, middle and posterior, all needing individual attention).
ACTIVITY	• The amount of activity a muscle generates also needs to be considered. Muscles inactive in everyday living may need a greater volume of work in the gym.
INTENSITY	• How hard or intense is the effort put into each rep and set will affect the volume of work in a workout session.

Figure 10.2 Segment motion points (biceps muscle) (a) short head (lower aspect) A–B (b) long head (lower aspect) A–B
(c) short head (upper aspect) A–B (d) long head (upper aspect) A–B

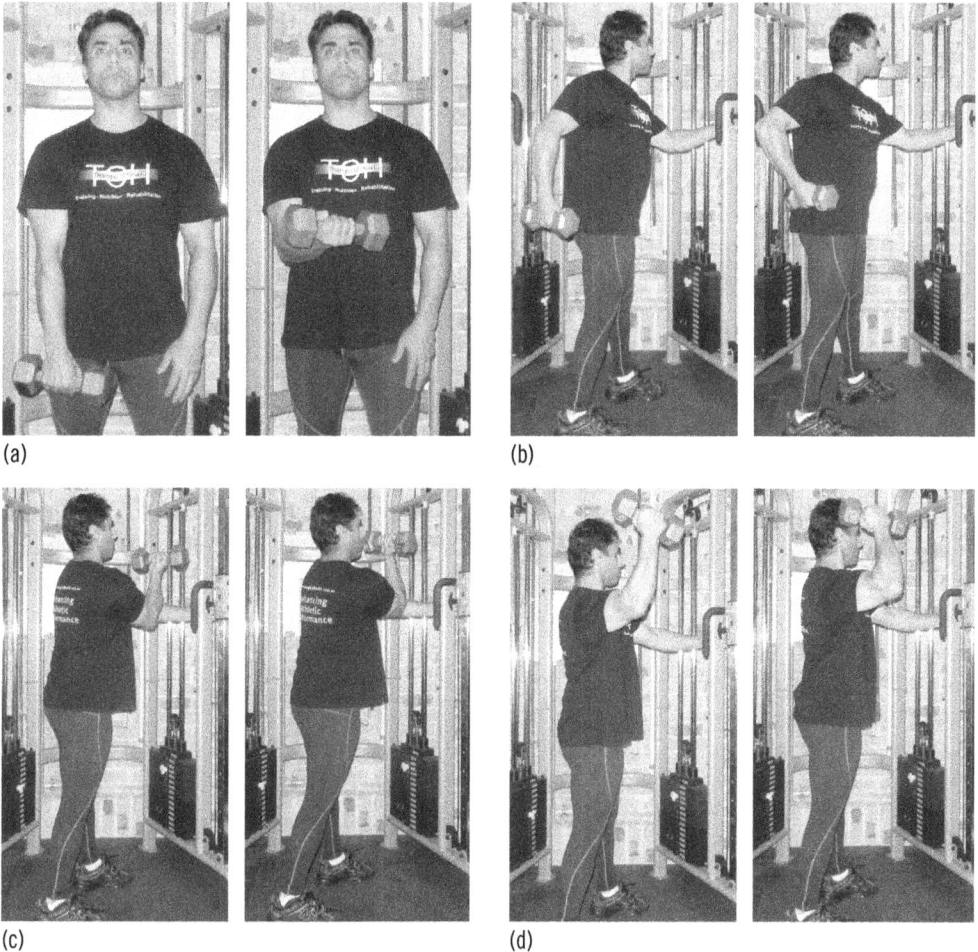

(a)

(b)

(c)

(d)

Working Weight

Unilateral training requires a totally different mindset when determining working weight for a prime moving muscle, especially for people who have trained in a bilateral fashion for many years and are conditioned to using large amounts of weight.

Determining an appropriate weight is best gauged using common sense; namely, executing an exercise with a specific muscle using a light and realistic weight that will allow the muscle to contract for a nominated number of repetitions. Using this simple method creates a reference point for strength that can be used as a guide.

This common-sense approach of gauging weight must continue with each rep, set, exercise and muscle as energy levels change. Changes in strength and performance will either decrease or increase. Generally, as a workout progresses and energy sources are used, the common effect will be decreased strength and effort.

On the other hand, strength can sometimes increase as a workout progresses, possibly due to a lack of initial warming up and inhibited blood flow, limiting energy to muscles at the early stages of a workout.

Irrespective of the progression point during a workout, strength levels of the prime moving muscle must be continuously catered for. This is best achieved by determining the weight of the next set at the conclusion of the preceding set, as each completed set will result in a degree of exhaustion or increased energy levels.

(*Note:* To safeguard against injury, any increase of resistance weight for a prime moving muscle should be carried out in small and realistic increments.)

Rest between Exercises and Sets

Rest periods during unilateral training differ greatly from those for traditional bilateral training. Training in a unilateral manner automatically reduces the weight that can be used, and the intensity generated by the body as a whole. This expedites the recovery of muscles between exercises and sets, subsequently decreasing rest periods.

Ways to gauge rest requirements include analysing breathing patterns, energy levels, focus and concentration. Breathing heavily is a good indication that the body is still recovering; normal breathing is a sign that the body is ready to resume exercise. Energy levels, high or low, will affect focus, concentration and the desire to proceed.

An important and unique aspect of unilateral training that must be taken into consideration is this: while one prime moving muscle is working, the reciprocal muscle on the other side of the body is resting.

Ultimately, recovery time and rest periods will vary from person to person, which makes a common-sense approach ideal.

The following variables will affect rest time:

- anaerobic/aerobic conditioning
- energy levels
- illness
- temperature
- extent of social networking (that is, extent to which one chats, uses mobile phone etc. between sets).

'Rest: take it if you feel you need it.'

How Hard?

How hard? relates to intensity, the effort or exertion made by a prime moving muscle against a resistance during an exercise. Simply put, it's how hard you train.

What level of intensity is appropriate for a person is, has been and always will be, contentious among those who engage in resistance training exercise.

To show intensity, some people will scream, shout, grunt, drop and throw weights, even hit each other or the equipment, viewing this as a rite of passage. Others believe that muscle soreness at the end of a training session is a means of gauging training intensity, imperative in achieving their goals.

A common-sense approach is once again required when determining intensity, as personal drive in pursuing goals can sometimes cloud one's judgement, making one lose sight of what is productive, healthy and logical in the long term.

Ultimately, the individual person must decide this issue, dictated by his or her wants, needs, level of experience and specific goals.

Creating Intensity

The first and most obvious way to create intensity for a prime moving muscle is by increasing the weight to one to which the muscle is unaccustomed.

This option requires vigilance so that the focus stays on contracting the prime moving muscle in a controlled manner, safeguarding against accelerated momentum and possible injury.

Sometimes injury may dictate the need to find other means of creating intensity (for example, by increasing volume, decreasing rest or using alternating exercises and so on). Increased volume means either a higher number of repetitions or sets or a combination of both, while decreased rest time between sets and exercises increases the work rate of not only the prime moving muscle but also the body as a whole.

Specific types of repetitions, such as forced and negative repetitions, are also viable options for increasing or creating intensity.

Measuring Intensity

Resistance training intensity can be measured by either analysing the percentage of one repetition maximum (that is, lifting the maximum weight possible with one muscle contraction) or a perceived scale of effort.

The most common (and standard) way of measuring resistance training intensity is by working the muscle at a percentage of one repetition maximum (or 1RM). This entails executing a muscle contraction of a particular exercise with the heaviest weight possible for a single repetition. Ideally, finding out a 1RM should be carried out with the muscle contracting and moving the nominated weight in a smooth and controlled manner, not using tremendous effort, which can increase the risk of injury.

The amount of weight raised for a single repetition will then create a reference point for gauging intensity.

- For example, executing one repetition with 20 kilograms for a dumbbell curl would constitute working at 100% of 1RM, while executing it with 15 kilograms would be 75% of 1RM.

Using this method to gauge intensity necessitates a reference point for 1RM of every exercise used, a task that can increase the risk of injury and that will change periodically.

A perceived scale of effort is another way of gauging intensity, using the numbers 1–10 to represent minimum and maximum muscle exertion, respectively. A perceived scale is highly recommended as a means of gauging resistance training intensity and one that is unique for individual needs and capabilities.

Over-training

A fine line exists between intensity and over-training. Potential consequences of over-training are fatigue, exhaustion, poor recovery and apathy. Regular high-intensity training will ultimately produce an over-trained state and malfunctioning of the body. For long-term health benefits and goal efficiency, high-intensity resistance training should be kept to a minimum.

Table 10.3: Over-training: signs and symptoms.

SIGNS	SYMPTOMS
Weight loss	Appetite loss
Deflated muscles	Apathy
Tired appearance	Lethargy
Muscle tightness	Tension/anxiety

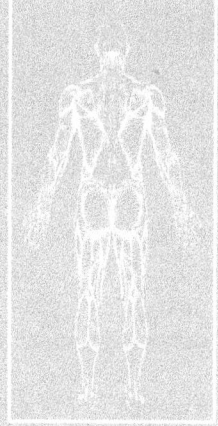

11
BMC Training System Equipment

T he majority of exercises that make up the BMC Training System revolve around the use of dumbbells and cable-pulley machines.

This chapter outlines the benefits of using these machines. Dumbbells and cable-pulley machines are versatile weight resistance tools that best accommodate the biomechanics and natural curvilinear movement patterns created by the human body.

(*Note:* Although some exercises described in Section Four are executed on linear machines, their restrictive nature is overcome by addressing movement pattern components such as position and motion.)

'The BMC Training System is a reality: don't hide from it. Embrace it!'

Dumbbell and Cable-pulley Machines – Benefits

Unilateral training, which involves isolating a prime moving muscle and its aspects, is the cornerstone of the BMC Training System. The system's integral partners are the dumbbell and adjustable cable-pulley machines.

It is these specific resistance tools that allow the hands, feet, related limbs and joints to be placed in varying positions and angles (to varying degrees) to create an efficient and near-perfect muscle contraction, while lessening the stress on, and potential risk of injury to, joints and muscles.

The dumbbell and cable-pulley machines best accommodate the natural curvilinear line of a muscle contraction. They also assist in fighting both the force of gravity and inertia by enabling a prime moving muscle to be conveniently placed in a maximised leverage position.

Although both pieces of equipment offer similar benefits, cable-pulley machines have some advantages over the dumbbell, such as position and stability in certain exercises.

Adjustable cable-pulley machines are designed so that the pulley can be adjusted, allowing it to be placed in a position that negates the force of gravity. This creates a smoother and more stable muscle contraction. For example, a biceps exercise using a dumbbell with the arm flexed at the shoulder joint requires greater focus and stability than if it were carried out on a cable-pulley machine (Figure 11.1).

(*Note:* Gravity plays a major role in mechanical advantage during resistance exercise; the further away a resistance weight is located from the body, the less strength and leverage a muscle has.)

Figure 11.1 (a) Cable-pulley biceps curl (b) Dumbbell biceps curl

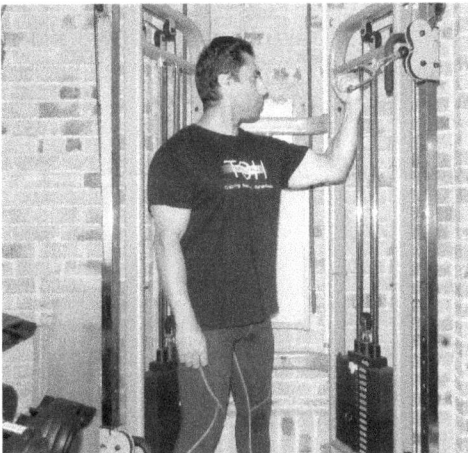

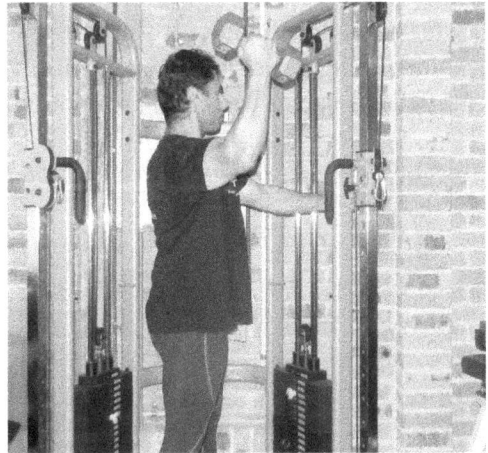

(a)   (b)

Negative Effects of the Barbell

The other key factor with the BMC Training System is the absence of probably the most famous and widely used piece of equipment in the world – the barbell.

Those who use the barbell believe that it is a superior exercise apparatus looked upon in the world of resistance training as the benchmark for the creation of power, strength and muscular size.

This is a misconception, reflecting a limited understanding or knowledge of anatomy, physiology and biomechanics (but, nonetheless, a view that has been ingrained in our culture for decades).

The reasons why a barbell should not be used to carry out any form of resistance exercise are detailed below:

- It is a linear piece of equipment that does not cater to the natural movement patterns of the body.

- It allows unrealistic amounts of weight to be used for a prime moving muscle.

- It increases the likelihood of accelerated momentum being used.

- It is a restrictive piece of equipment, placing prime moving muscles and joints in awkward, unnatural positions. This affects normal biomechanics.

- It restricts resistance being distributed equally between a prime moving muscle on one side of the body and its equivalent muscle on the other side.

- It leads to poor muscle development, a result of a barbell's limitations in contracting various aspects of a prime moving muscle (Figure 11.2).

- It decreases awareness of muscle weakness and imbalance, subsequently concealing slow deterioration of a muscle and increasing the possibility of impending injuries through a compensatory process.

- It is unable to effectively cater to varying muscles with a common joint action. (Figure 8.1(c)).

(*Note:* Here's a question for those who currently engage in weight-bearing resistance exercise: Do you suffer from chronic neck, shoulder, lower back, elbow, wrist, hip or knee joint pain? If the answer is 'yes' to any of these, look at the barbell as being a potential source of these problems.)

Figure 11.2 (a) The barbell is restricting placement of the biceps long head in a lengthened position. (b) No such restriction exists with the dumbbell.

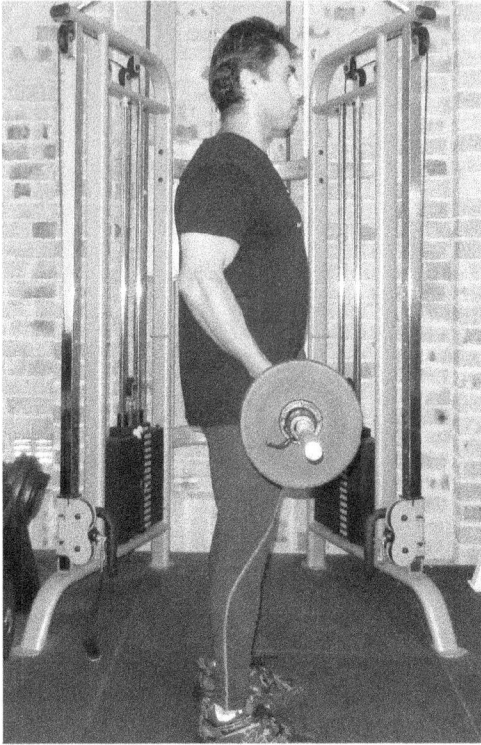

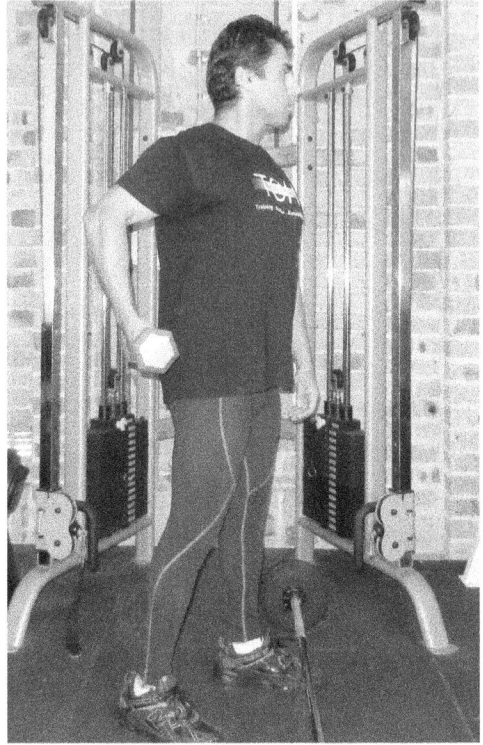

(a)

(b)

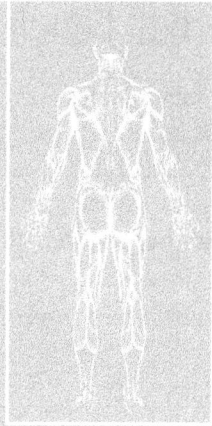

12
Compound Exercises
– Why Avoid Them?

To this point in Section Three, the components of unilateral training have been explained, outlining the arguments for, and the benefits of, this approach to resistance training. This section would not be complete, however, without reiterating why unilateral training is endorsed over compound bilateral training.

This chapter focuses on the faults, negative aspects and dangers of the most commonly used compound exercises for bilateral resistance training – traditionally, the barbell squat, bench press, deadlift, military press and biceps curl. Each of these exercises is designed as the ultimate exercise for a specific area or muscle of the body. The squat benefits the legs; the bench press, the chest; deadlifts, the back; the military press, the shoulders; and the barbell curl, the biceps.

There is no doubt that these exercises do a great job in building muscle mass, power and strength; unfortunately, they do so at a cost to the body.

Outlined below are the unproductive and unnatural movement patterns, as well as the potential dangers, created by using the barbell for the following exercises: bench press, squat, deadlift, military press and biceps curl.

'The truth may hurt temporarily but the pain of injury may last a lifetime.'

Barbell bench press

The bench press is an upper body exercise. It is traditionally carried out by lying on a flat bench and raising the barbell. It is probably the most recognised and popular resistance training exercise in the world, commonly seen as the best way to develop the pectoralis major muscles, or chest muscles; many regard it as the benchmark of gauging the power, strength and dominance of the upper body in the supine position. It is typical that when the topic of weight resistance training arises in a conversation the question is 'How much do ya bench?'

It is automatic to assume that a bench press exercise engages the chest muscles; in reality, execution of the exercise also recruits the triceps and anterior deltoid muscles.

Unfortunately, the barbell bench press is also very much an exercise that appeals to the ego; it falls short in developing the chest muscles in an efficient and safe manner.

Reasons why the barbell bench press exercise (Figure 12.1) should be avoided:

* The barbell bench press restricts the natural movement pattern of the contracting chest muscles, placing the wrist, elbow and shoulder joints in awkward and dangerous positions; in turn, this puts stress and pressure on the attachment points of the muscles and associated soft tissue structures involved.

* The linear or straight-line nature of the barbell requires hands to be placed in a position that increases the likelihood of the upper arm jamming into the AC joint (the joint where the outer or lateral aspect of the collarbone meets the shoulder blade). This problem magnifies when the exercise is executed on an inclined bench.

* Focus on the adduction (of the arms) function of the chest muscles can be lost, due to the assistance of the shoulder (anterior deltoid) and triceps muscles during the exercise.

* A much more serious problem occurs when people grab the bar of the barbell with a thumbless grip (that is, the thumb is positioned under, instead of over, the bar). This creates two dangerous and problematic scenarios: firstly, it is harder to balance the bar holding it this way and, secondly, it forces the wrist joints into hyper-extension, increasing the risk of damage to the median nerve.

Figure 12.1(a) Barbell bench press (front profile)

Start:

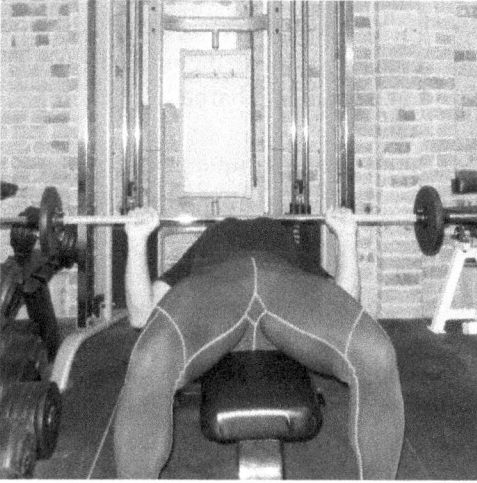

Finish:

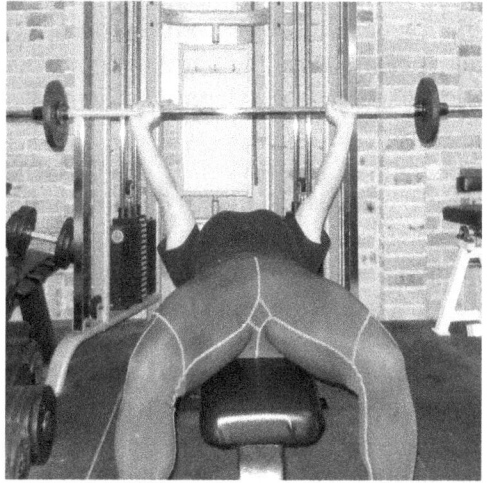

Figure 12.1(b) Barbell bench press (side profile)

Start:

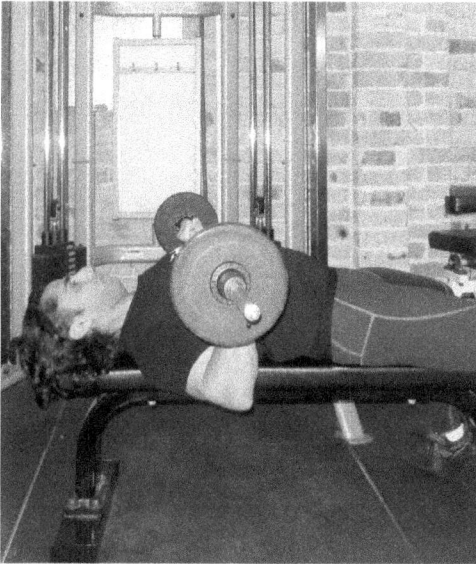

Finish:

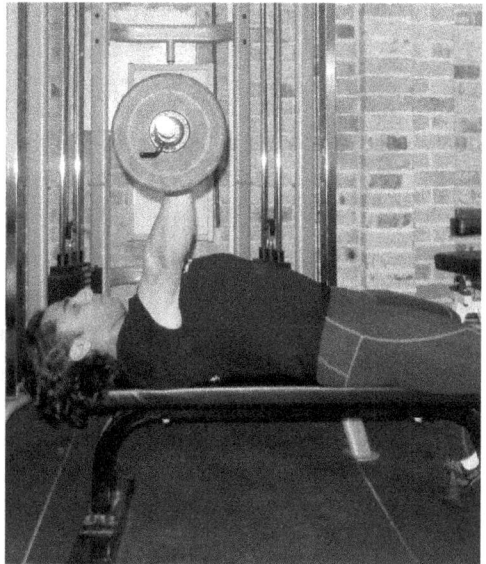

Barbell squat

The squat is a lower body exercise. It is traditionally carried out by raising the barbell from a squatting position. Its purpose is to develop the thigh muscles, specifically the quadriceps. Of all the traditional compound exercises (of those mentioned earlier), the squat enables the largest amount of weight to be used on a barbell.

Compared with the other compound exercises, the squat is unique in its execution: the barbell is in contact with the body, positioned to the rear, and sitting across the back of the shoulders. All the other compound exercises require grabbing or gripping the barbell for their execution. The squat also requires gripping the barbell but this is done only to provide stability, not to execute the exercise.

Advocates of the squat exercise argue that squatting is a natural movement carried out in everyday living, such as by sitting down or picking up something off the ground. This is true, but these simple acts are not carried out with a weight across the shoulders to the rear of the body.

As much as the barbell squat is touted for being a great quadriceps exercise, a large part of the exercise is carried out through the hips and lower back muscles. To verify this, compare the amount of weight used for a barbell squat with that for a leg extension exercise. The weight used during a leg extension exercise (which isolates only the quadricep muscles) is a fraction of the weight used during the squat exercise.

The negative aspects of the barbell squat encompass issues relating to the shoulders, neck, spine and knees (to name a few body parts).

Reasons why the barbell squat exercise (Figure 12.2) should be avoided:

- Individual bones (known as the vertebrae) that make up the spine vary in shape, size and density; they start off as small bones at the top and progressively increase in size down the spine. During the squat exercise, the barbell sits on the delicate structures of the shoulder girdle (rear of the body) and on the first few vertebrae of the thoracic portion of the spine. Placing a large amount of weight on this area of the body (which the squat enables one to do) automatically increases pressure on the soft tissue structures (that help to stabilise the spine) such as the muscles, tendons, ligaments, nerve fibres and discs.

- Discs, or intervertebral discs as they are correctly known (which separate individual vertebrae), become less hydrated and more brittle as we age, increasing the chances of spinal damage and of developing back pain.

- The position of the barbell across the shoulder girdle automatically causes unnatural backward rotation (hyper-rotation) of the arms at the shoulder joints as well as awkward forward placement of the neck and head.

- Using the hands to maintain stability hyper-extends the hands at the wrist, increasing the risk of nerve damage in that region.

- Poor biomechanical function of the hip or back region (due to a genetic factor), or faulty muscle and/or nerve function, can cause the weight during the squat exercise to be distributed too far forward. This places pressure on the knees (which should function only as the pivoting point); the risk of injury is increased if too much weight is lifted.

- Deep-squatting, where thighs, moving past the parallel position, will stretch the patella tendon, can also be dangerous for other areas of the body, such as the lower back and hips.

- Poor flexibility in hip, knee and ankle regions increases forward movement of the upper body during the down-and-up phase of the exercise; this will generally increase the work load carried out by the back muscles, instead of the intended quadricep muscles.

- Contraction of the abdominal muscle is encouraged during the squat exercise on the assumption that this will protect the back during the exercise. At face value, this seems sensible. Unfortunately, this assumption contradicts the laws of physiology that relate to agonist and antagonist muscles; namely, that when one muscle contracts, the opposing muscle must relax. When the upper body requires extension during the ascending phase of the exercise, it will be carried out by the back muscles; this will be limited if the abdominal muscle (one muscle, though with multiple heads or origin attachments) is contracted, as it is the opposing muscle to the back muscles.

- A version of the barbell squat that some people execute is to squat on a bench or seat. The exercise is then carried out by squatting to the point where the hips and bench structure meet, stopping and then ascending. Stopping allows the hip muscles to relax when they should be tensing for the ascent; this automatically distributes the weight through the back, creating a dangerous scenario for potential back damage.

Figure 12.2 Barbell squat

Start: **Finish:**

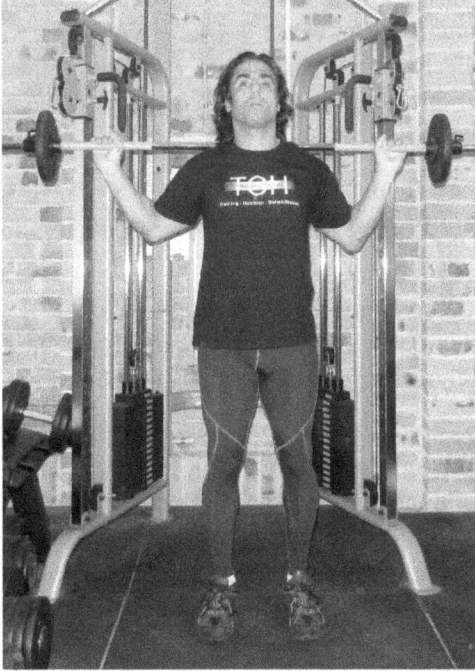 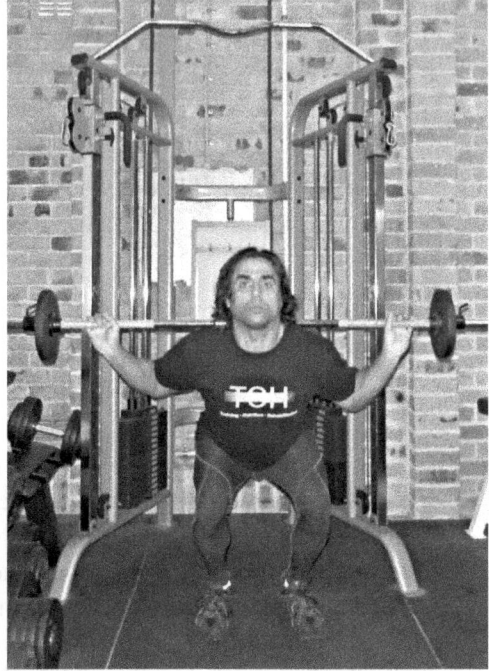

Barbell deadlift

The deadlift is an upper body exercise. It is traditionally carried out by raising the barbell off the ground from a squatting position. Its purpose is to develop the back muscles that run along the spine.

The deadlift for many people is an intimidating, frightening exercise. The fear stems from the belief that it will injure the lower back. Hence many are deterred from attempting it.

Reasons why the barbell deadlift exercise (Figure 12.3) should be avoided:

- A traditional barbell deadlift requires a person to hold the bar with one hand under and one hand over the bar. The 'hand over' is a pronated position, which relaxes the biceps muscle, while the 'hand under' is supinated, contracting the biceps. Placing the hands in an over/under position changes the alignment of the arms, shoulders, back and hips, automatically creating abnormal angles and structural imbalance, and increasing the risk of injury and poor muscle development.

- To try to alleviate problem issues relating to the traditional deadlift, some choose an alternative version, one where both hands grip the barbell in a pronated (palms facing backward) position. This rectifies issues related to the shoulder and biceps, but it then positions the barbell further away from the body, creating a mechanical disadvantage and decreasing the safety of the exercise during its execution.

- Some people tend to hyper-extend at the end of the exercise. This can make the back vulnerable to injury.

Figure 12.3 Barbell deadlift

Start: **Finish:**

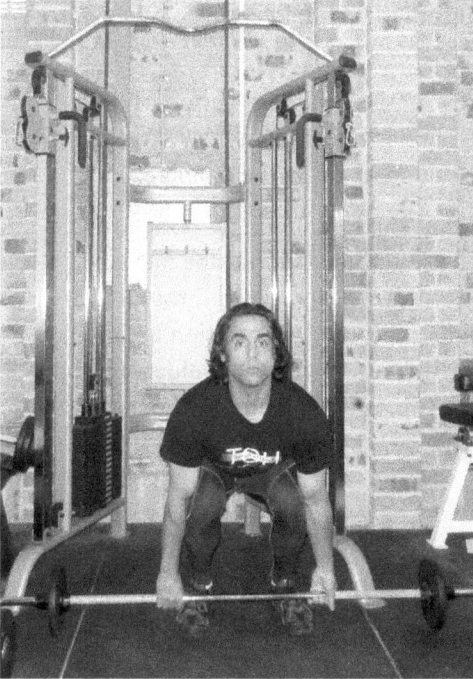

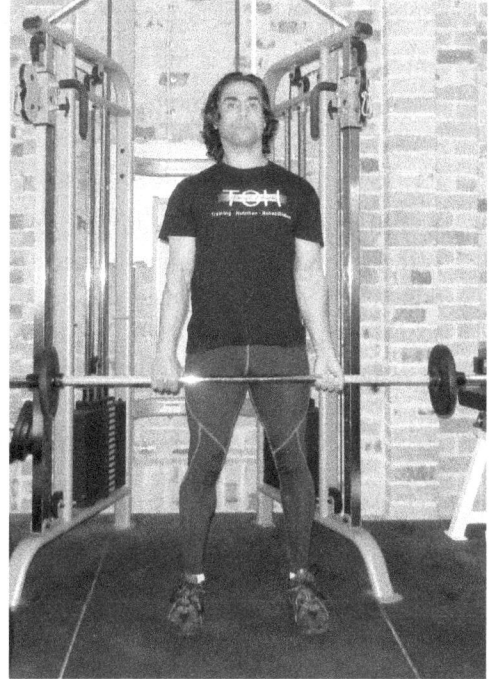

Barbell military press

The barbell military press is an exercise traditionally carried out by raising the barbell above the head from a standing position. The sole purpose of this exercise is to develop the shoulder muscles, specifically the deltoids. It is another compound movement that allows large amounts of weight to be used.

Some think that the military press develops the whole deltoid muscle; this is impossible as the deltoid muscle is made up of three different portions, each with a differing function.

Reasons why the barbell military press exercise (Figure 12.4) should be avoided:

- Executing the military press distributes excessive weight through the lower back, increasing lumbar curvature, and making the lower back vulnerable to injury.

- The explosive nature of the exercise makes it tempting to use accelerated momentum, created through recruiting muscles such as the arms, legs and hips in raising the weight. This increases the risk of injury to the elbow and shoulder joints and to their respective connective tissues.

- A tendency for the triceps muscles to carry out most of the movement removes the emphasis on the deltoid muscles, thus creating weakness through a lack of development.

- The linear nature of the barbell, coupled with the awkward nature of the exercise, affects joints such as the wrists, placing them in hyper-extended positions. Once again, this increases the potential for nerve damage.

- A different version to the military press that is popular among bodybuilders is the barbell press behind the neck. It is an exercise that has the barbell positioned behind the head and neck, with movement created through the arms at the shoulder joints. Problems that stem from this position are created by the arms being placed in a hyper-rotated position at the shoulder joint; this causes the humeral head and neck to slide forward – a dangerous position that stretches ligaments and the anterior portion of the deltoid.

Figure 12.4 Barbell military press

Start: **Finish:**

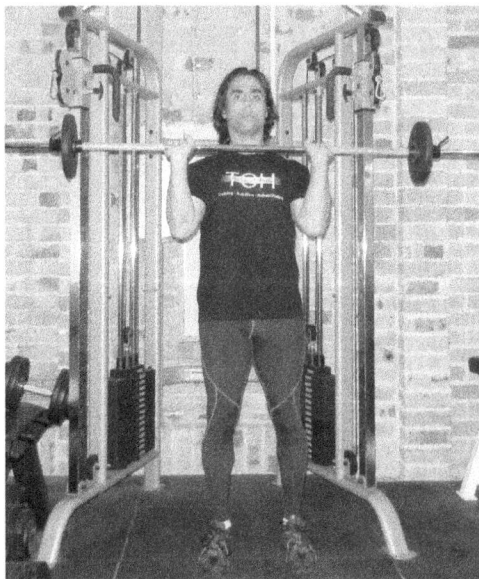 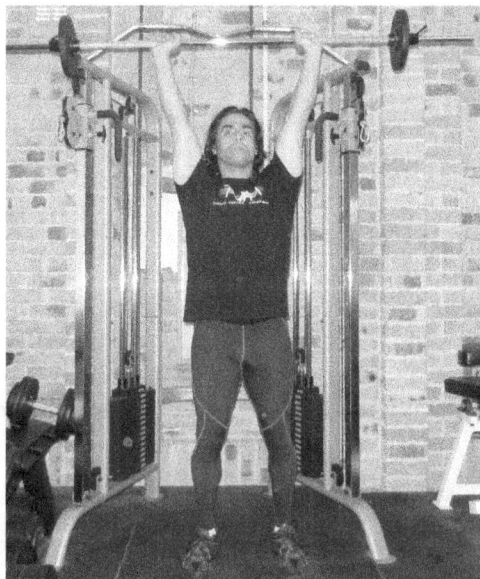

Barbell biceps curl

The biceps curl is an exercise traditionally carried out by raising the barbell in a curling action from a standing position. The purpose of the exercise is to develop the arm muscles, specifically the biceps. It is the most recognised arm exercise in the world.

Reasons why the biceps barbell curl exercise (Figure 12.5) should be avoided:

- It creates an unnatural position of the hands, which subsequently affects wrist, shoulder and elbow joints, and restricts the efficient and natural movement pattern of the contracting biceps muscles.

- The nature of the barbell restricts extension of the arm at the shoulder joint (Figure 11.2 (a)), subsequently stopping the long head of the biceps from being contracted in its most lengthened position.

- It is an exercise synonymous with use of accelerated momentum.

Figure 12.5 Barbell biceps curl

Start: **Finish:**

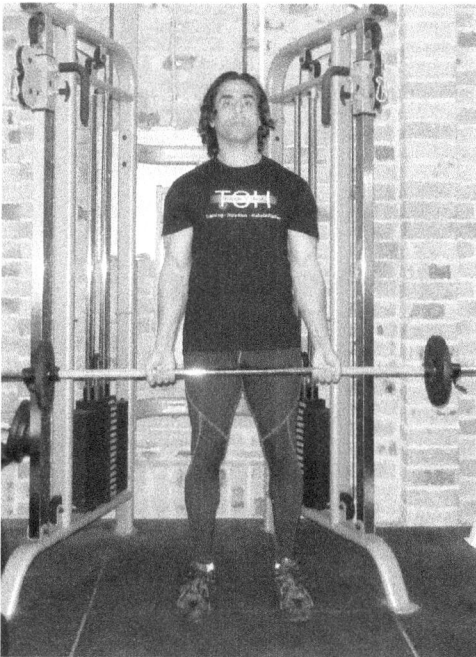 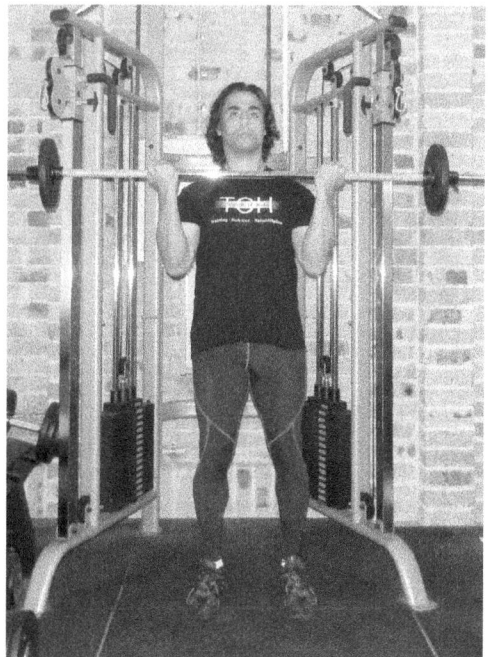

Table 12.1: Soft tissue injuries sustained by professional bodybuilders during traditional bilateral training with the barbell.

NAME	SOFT TISSUE INJURY	EXERCISE
Dorian Yates[1]	Biceps (left) Triceps (left) Fascia (right hip)	Reverse grip bent over row Pull over press Squat
Marcus Rhul[2]	Triceps (left)	Bench press
Jean-Pierre Fux[3]	Quadricep (left) Patella ligament (right)	Squat
Francis Bendatto[4]	Chest (right)	Bench press
Victor Martinez[5]	Chest (left)	Bench press
Branch Warren[6]	Biceps (right)	Curl
Tony Freeman[7]	Chest (right)	Bench press
Achim Albrecht[8]	Biceps (left)	Preacher curl
Kevin Levrone[9]	Chest (right)	Bench press
Berry DeMey[10]	Chest (right)	Bench press
Rich Gaspari[11]	Chest (left)	Incline press (Smith machine)

Sources:
1. Robson D 2008. 6-time Mr Olympia: Dorian Yates interview – now famous 1993 gym shots, injuries and current affairs. Bodybuilding.com: Meridian, USA. Viewed 6 September 2010, <http://www.bodybuilding.com/fun/dorian_yates_interview_1993_gym_shots.htm>; Yates D 2010. Blood & guts: breaking the rules for big wheels. Muscular Development 47(8):318; Yates D 2010. Blood & guts: Mr Olympia memories. Muscular Development 47(10):298,300.

2. Harris R 2007. Part 3 - Branch and Markus fire off their large caliber guns. Muscular Development 44(9):236.

3. Jean-Pierre Fux squat accident. Intense Muscle: USA. Viewed 6 September 2010, <http://www.intensemuscle.com/showthread.php?t=20109>.

4. Benfatto F & Team Flex 2007. The real Francis Benfatto: the life and times of a bodybuilding superstar. Part 2: Flex (Australian edn). July/August. p. 52.

5. Muscular Development: USA. Viewed 7 July 2010, <http://forums.musculardevelopment.com/showthread.php?t=56627&page=17>.

6. Warren B 2010. Mass with class: the Texas titan. Muscular Development 47(12):338–42.

7. Merritt G 2007. Freeman's back story. Flex (Australian edn). September/October. p. 32.

8. Albrecht A 1993. My torn biceps. EBSCO Host Connection: USA. Viewed 19 September 2013, <http://connection.ebscohost.com/c/articles/9312213363/my-torn-biceps>.

9. Hilson, Jr R 1994. Built to win. The Baltimore Sun: Baltimore, USA. Viewed 19 September 2013, <http://articles.baltimoresun.com/1994-07-03/features/1994184218_1_kevin-levrone-glen-burnie-time-to-eat/3>.

10. McGough P 2013. Berry De Mey: a Dutch master – the day his dream died. Muscular Development: USA. Viewed 19 September 2013, <http://www.musculardevelopment.com/team-md-blogs/the-mcgough-report/11830-berry-demey-a-dutch-master-the-day-his-dream-died-by-peter-mcgough.html#.Ud2Y323-tec/>.

11. Gaspari R 2012. The dragonslayer: how I tore my pec – a cautionary tale. Muscular Development 49(9):274,276.

SECTION FOUR

BMC Training
System Exercises

The equipment used in resistance training plays a pivotal role in dictating what type of movement pattern can be created.

In a bid to alleviate user compatibility issues, companies develop machines with multiple adjustment points to match individual body shapes and sizes. However, with the exception of dumbbells and adjustable cable-pulley machines, most machines, including barbells, come up short in matching the natural biomechanics of the human body.

Each and every exercise in the BMC Training System has been created with a specific goal in mind: to isolate a prime moving muscle and execute its function in the most natural and uninhibited movement pattern.

To those who are familiar with traditional bilateral resistance training, the appearance of some exercises in this section may look and seem unorthodox at times. Hopefully, this will not discourage their use for they offer many productive benefits.

'Nothing worthwhile in life is ever achieved without dedication, determination and discipline.'

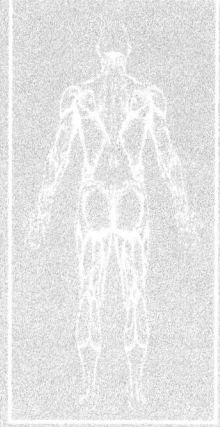

13
Unilateral Exercise for the Prime Moving Muscle

Whether you are familiar with resistance training or not, the BMC Training System will be a rewarding experience, or a unique change. Time and patience are paramount so that the mind and body can adapt to this change, especially for those not familiar with anatomy, physiology and resistance exercise.

The exercises in this chapter are a small sample of the many developed for the BMC Training System. These exercises have been designed to remove the guesswork about how to develop, strengthen and condition a prime moving muscle and its various aspects.

The exercises have been designed for execution in an extended or bent-limb fashion, catering to different muscle aspects, leverage and ROM so that the ultimate peak muscle contraction can be attained.

The advantages of straight or bent-limb position will depend on the prime moving muscle involved, the desired aspect and the specific exercise used, meaning that some muscles may produce a stronger and more efficient contraction in a bent-limb fashion than in a straight position, and vice versa.

It is important to remember that we are all different so an exact position or angle for one person may not be right for another. Practise and develop what is right for you.

'The BMC Training System exercises – short and sweet.'

(*Note:* To reduce risk of injury and improve athletic performance, it is important that, before any of the resistance exercises described in this chapter are undertaken, an appropriate amount of aerobic warming-up be conducted.

Also note the following precautions:

- Before using any structure to secure, stabilise or balance any part of the body during an exercise, check that it is secure, stable and sturdy.

- Do not grab any moving parts of a machine to stabilise yourself.

- Be aware that the capabilities of each muscle, its aspect and the particular exercise will be different.

- Consider the weight being used for resistance training: start with a light weight; then, if desired, the weight can be increased in small increments.

- The instructions for every exercise lists directions for only one prime moving muscle.

- The instructions need to be reversed when working the opposing prime moving muscle.

- Machines and/or equipment used to demonstrate exercises in this book may vary from those found in other environments.)

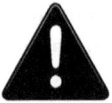

⚠ **Under no circumstances shall anyone aged under 18, anyone with mental or physical disadvantage or anyone who lacks experience in resistance weight training either attempt – or be encouraged to attempt – any of the exercises described in this book without the supervision of a qualified instructor.**

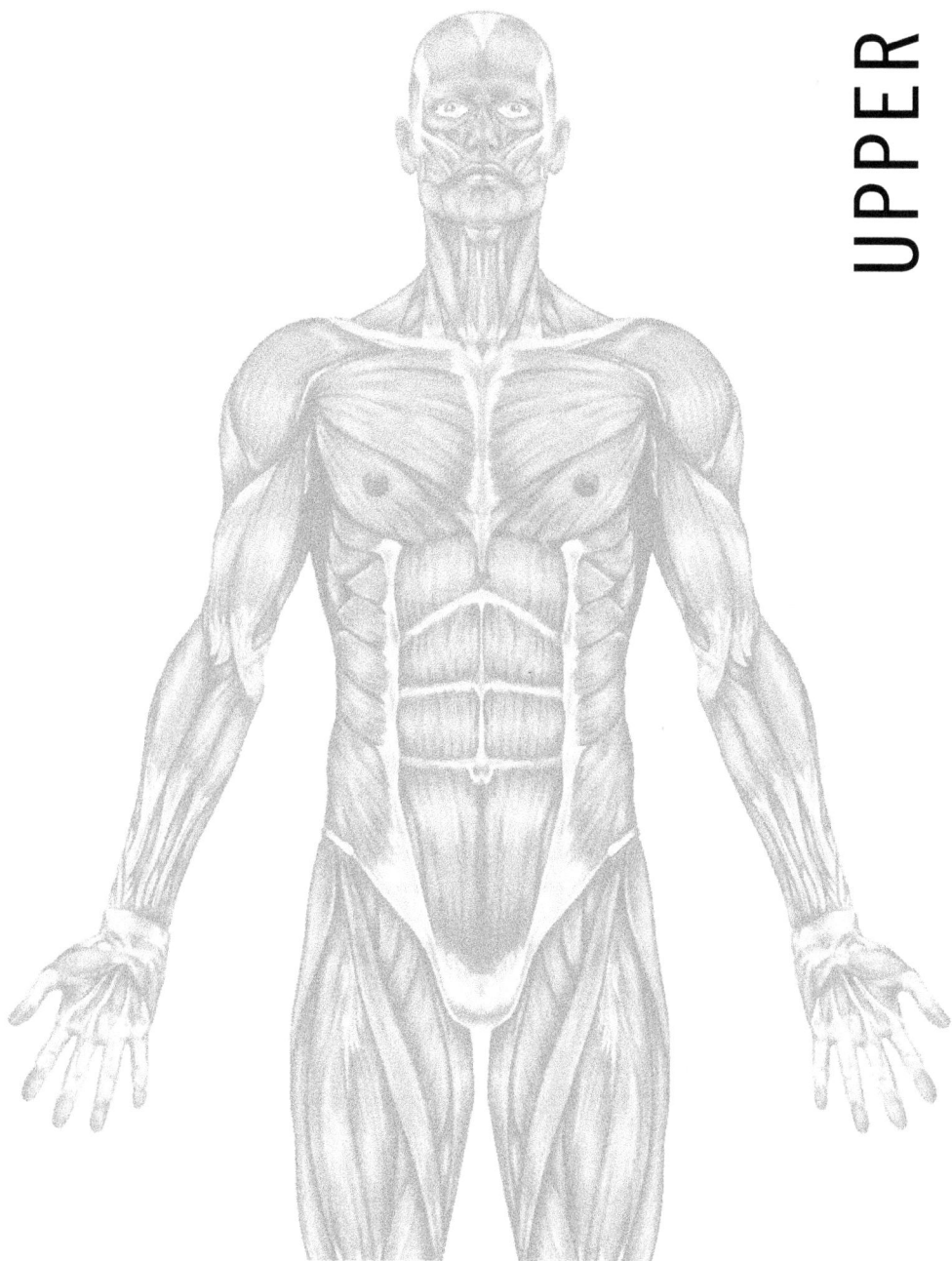

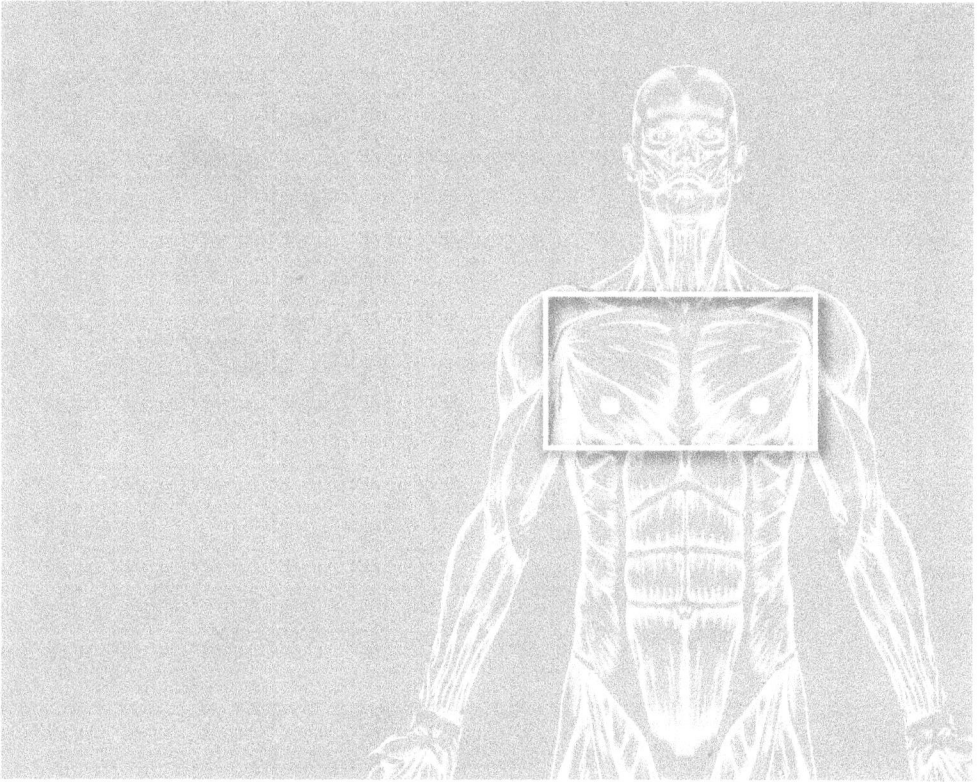

Chest Muscle Exercises

Pectoralis Major

The pectoralis major muscles (Figure 13.1), better known as the chest muscles, are made up of two heads: clavicular and sternocostal.

The 'pecs' as they are commonly called, function to adduct, flex and medially rotate the arm while also helping to maintain the arm and shoulder in a downward direction.

Figure 13.1 Pectoralis major muscle

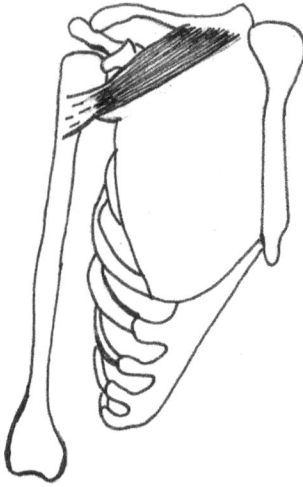

(a) clavicular head
(b) sternocostal head

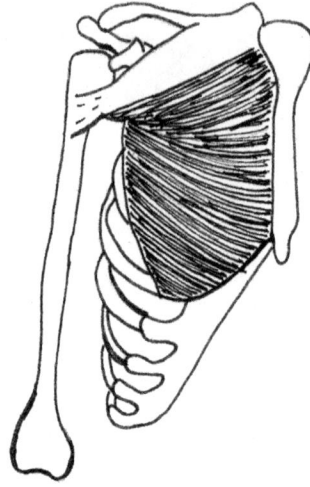

ORIGIN ATTACHMENT	INSERTION ATTACHMENT
• **Clavicle** (medial) • **Sternum** • **Ribs** (1 – 6) • **External oblique muscle**	• **Humerus** (bicipital groove)

Things to consider:

☑ Focus and execution of all exercises are via the shoulder joint.

☑ Minimise flexion or extension of elbow joint during exercises.

☑ Hand position for chest muscle exercises will be created via the elbow and shoulder joints.

DUMBBELL PRESS

Incline: Superior – Lateral Aspect

Start:

Lie on an incline bench (30–40°). Grab the dumbbell from below with the working hand and then **use both hands to raise it**. Secure opposing hand to a stable structure, and bend the working arm slightly at the elbow joint, grabbing the dumbbell with the working hand in a semi-prone position.

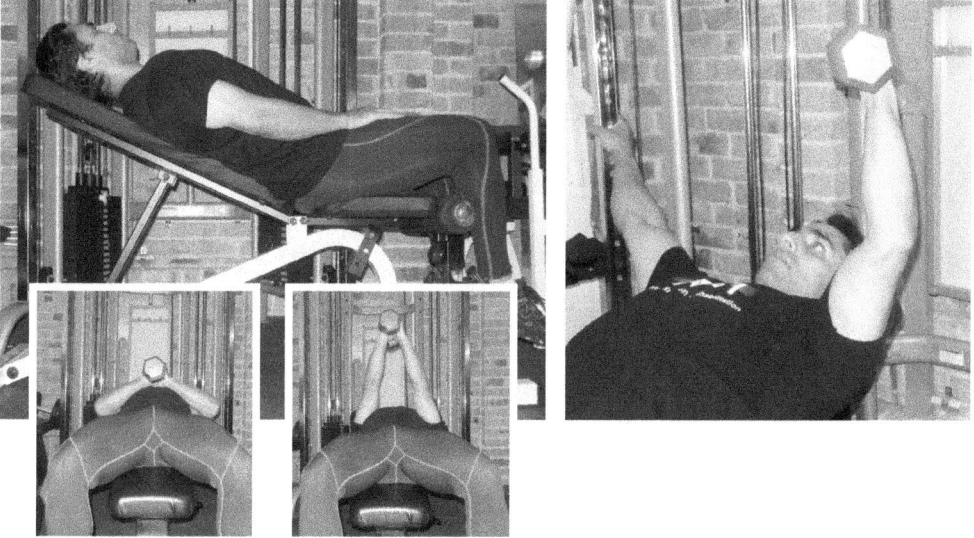

Raising dumbbell

Finish:

Adduct the working arm at the shoulder joint in a medial direction to initial contact of biceps and chest muscles.

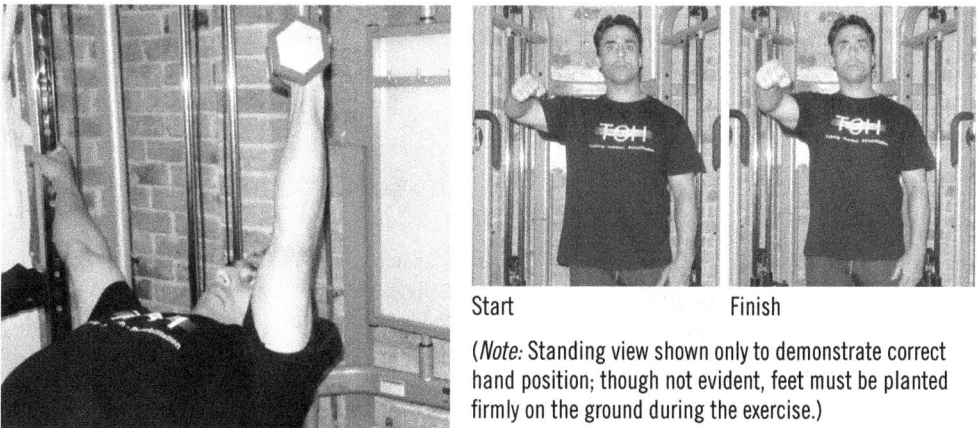

Start   Finish

(*Note:* Standing view shown only to demonstrate correct hand position; though not evident, feet must be planted firmly on the ground during the exercise.)

Supine: Middle – Lateral Aspect

Start:

Lie on a flat bench (180°). Grab the dumbbell from below with the working hand and then **use both hands to raise it**. Secure opposing hand to a stable structure, and bend the working arm slightly at the elbow joint, grabbing the dumbbell with the working hand in a semi-supine position.

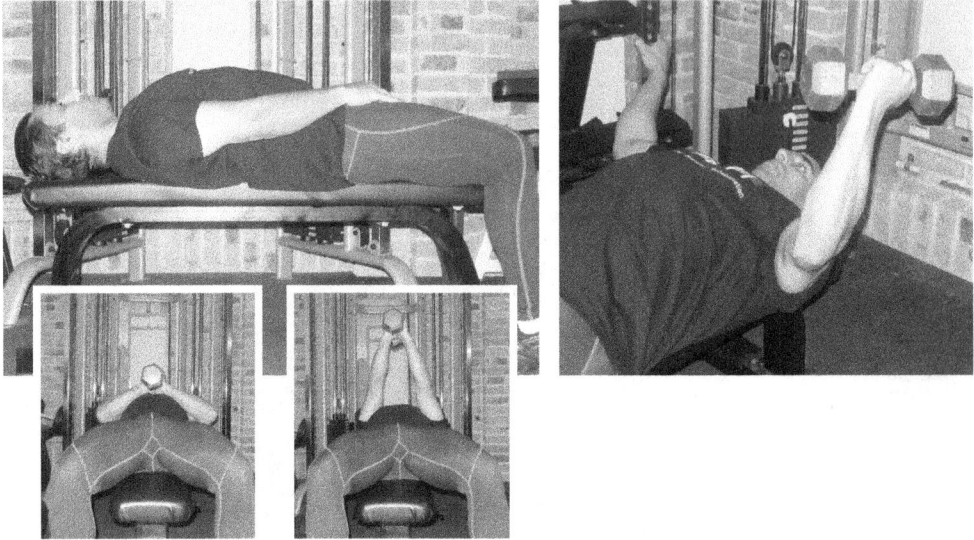

Raising dumbbell

Finish:

Adduct the working arm at the shoulder joint in a medial direction to initial contact of biceps and chest muscles.

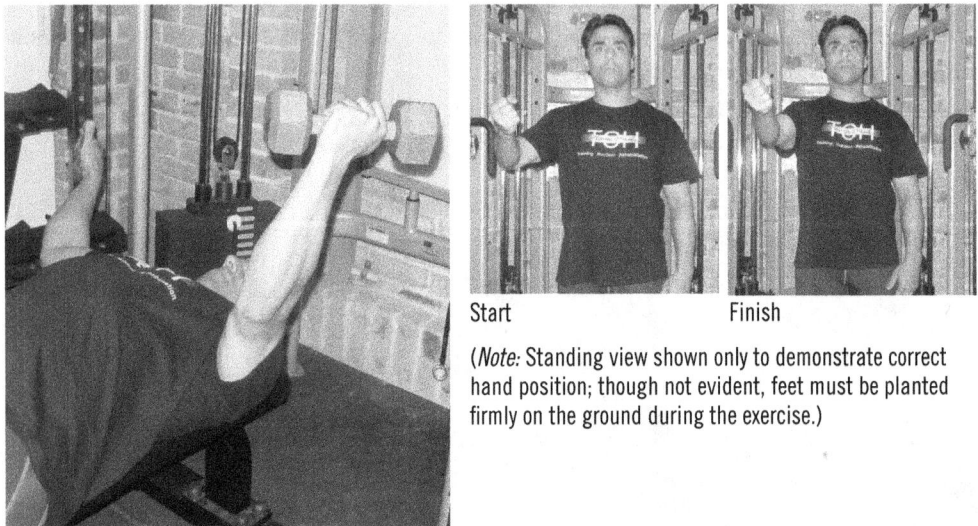

Start   Finish

(*Note:* Standing view shown only to demonstrate correct hand position; though not evident, feet must be planted firmly on the ground during the exercise.)

Decline: Inferior – Lateral Aspect

Start:

Lie on a decline bench (20–40°). Grab the dumbbell from below with the working hand and then **use both hands to raise it**. Secure opposing hand to a stable structure, and bend the working arm slightly at the elbow joint, grabbing the dumbbell with the working hand in a semi-prone position.

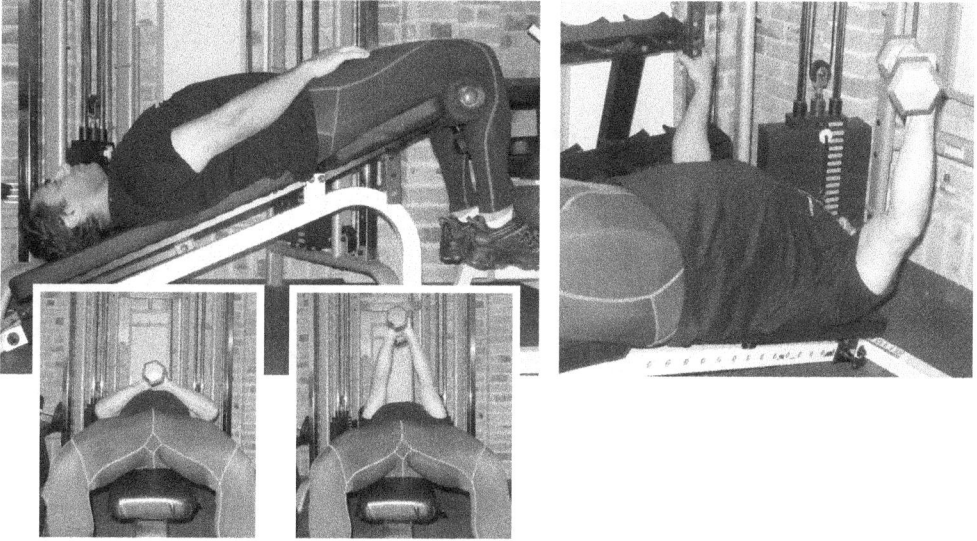

Raising dumbbell

Finish:

Adduct the working arm at the shoulder joint in a medial direction to initial contact of biceps and chest muscles.

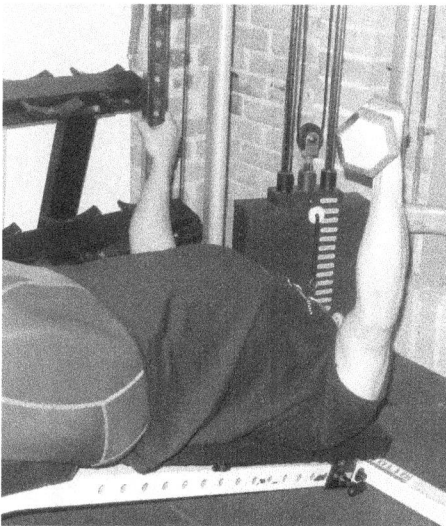

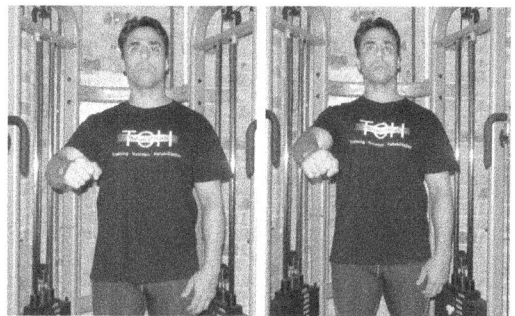

Start   Finish

(*Note:* Standing view shown only to demonstrate correct hand position; though not evident, feet must be secured to the machine or planted firmly on the ground during the exercise.)

CABLE-PULLEY ADDUCTOR/ROTATOR

Standing: Superior – Medial Aspect

Start:

Adopt a unilateral stance (see page 47 for an explanation). Securing the opposing hand to a stable structure, bend the working arm at approximately 90° and grab the stirrup handle, placing the working hand in a semi-prone position.

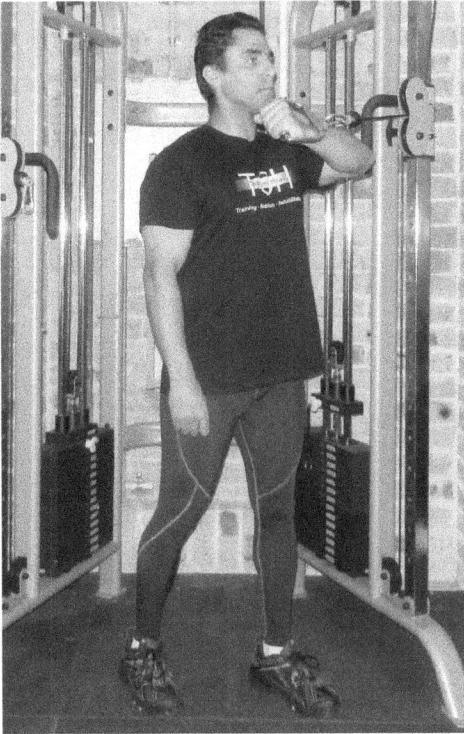

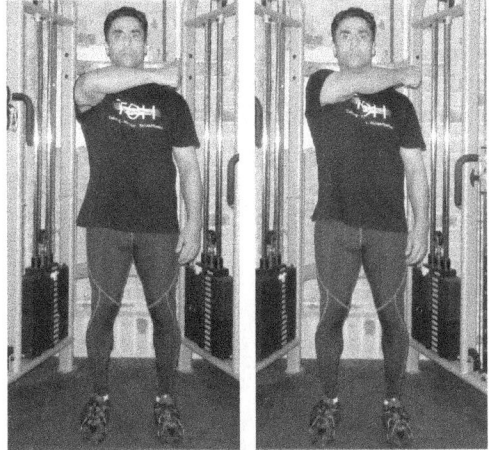

Front view

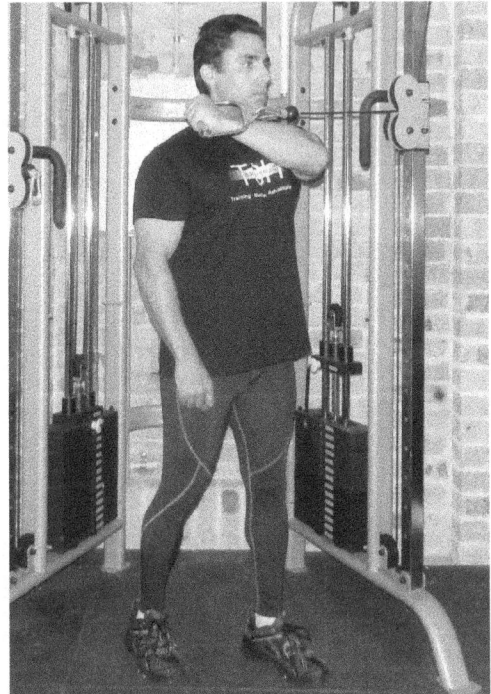

Finish:

Adduct and rotate the working arm at the shoulder joint in a medial direction to initial contact of biceps and chest muscles.

(*Note:* Though not evident in photographs, the opposing hand must be secured to a stable structure.)

Standing: Middle – Medial Aspect

Start:

Adopt a unilateral stance (see page 47 for an explanation). Securing the opposing hand to a stable structure, bend the working arm at approximately 90° and grab the stirrup handle, placing the working hand in a semi-supine position.

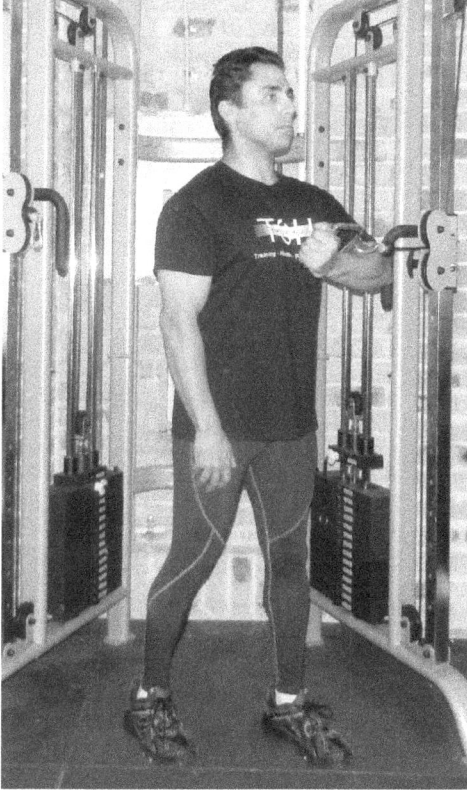

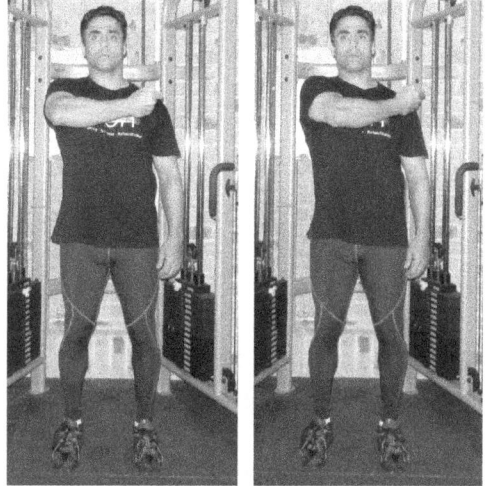

Front view

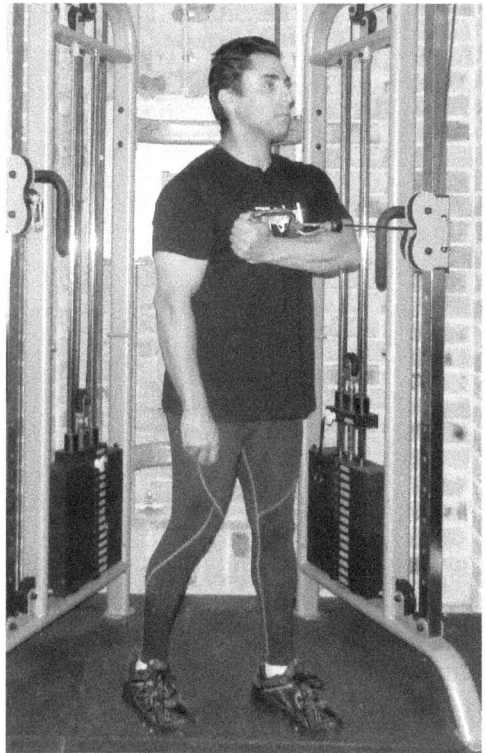

Finish:

Adduct and rotate the working arm at the shoulder joint in a medial direction to initial contact of biceps and chest muscles.

(*Note:* Though not evident in photographs, the opposing hand must be secured to a stable structure.)

Standing: Inferior – Medial Aspect

Start:

Adopt a unilateral stance (see page 47 for an explanation). Securing the opposing hand to a stable structure, bend the working arm at approximately 90° and grab the stirrup handle, placing the working hand in a semi-prone position.

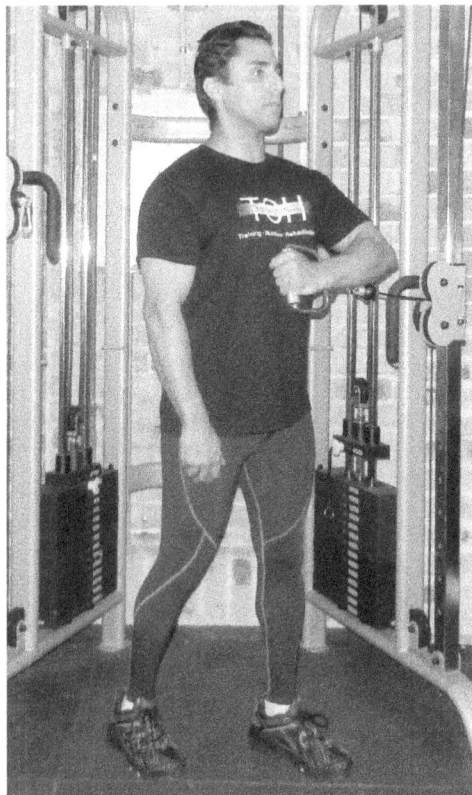

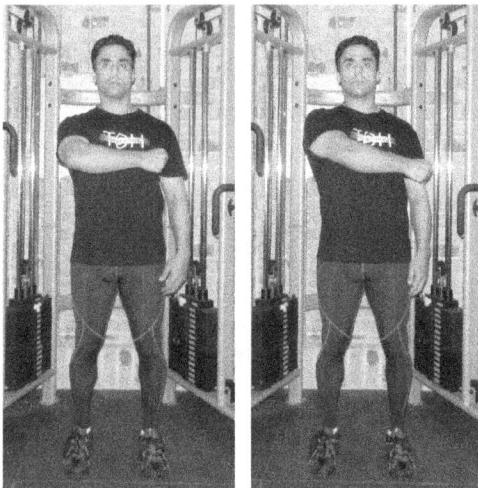

Front view

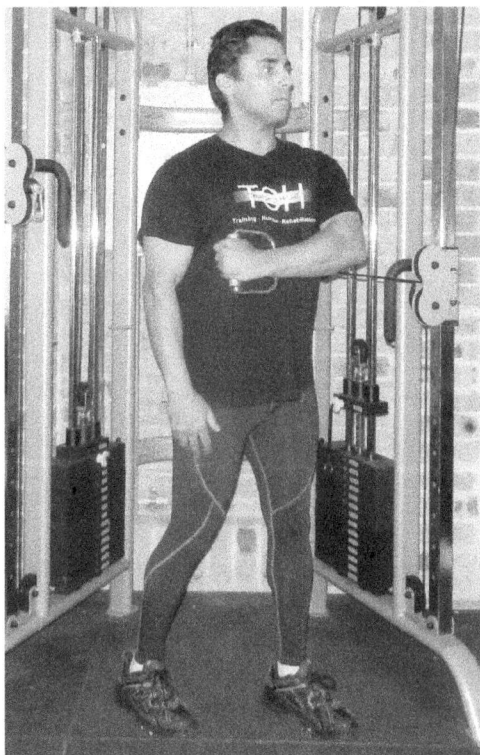

Finish:

Adduct and rotate the working arm at the shoulder joint in a medial direction to initial contact of biceps and chest muscles.

(*Note:* Though not evident in photographs, the opposing hand must be secured to a stable structure.)

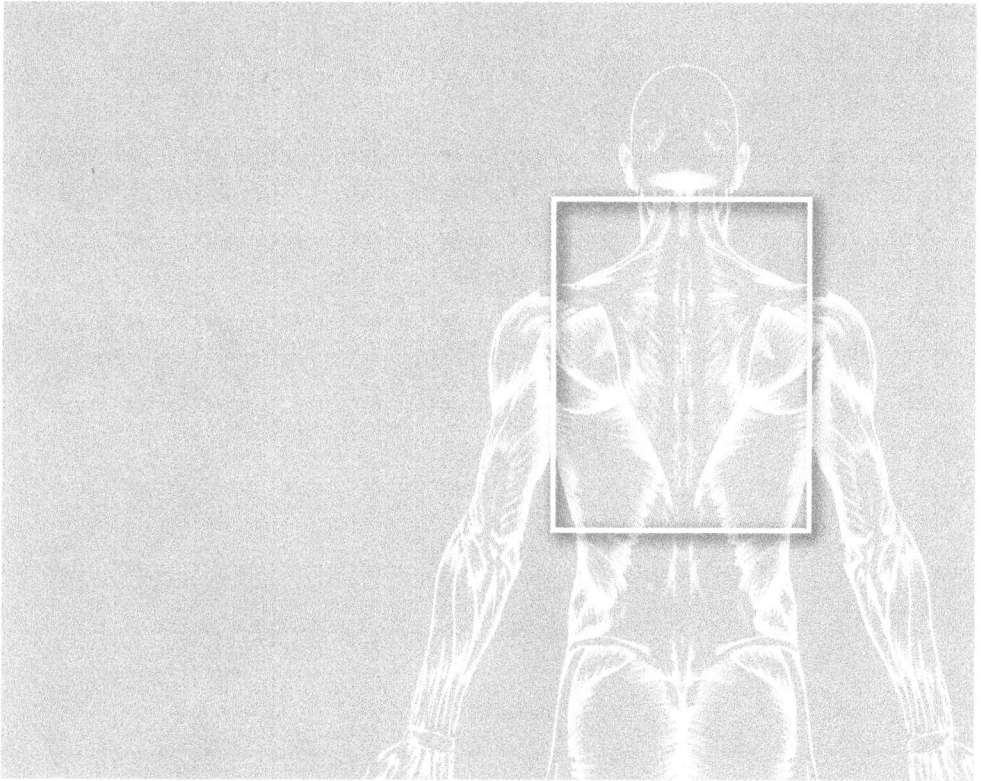

Trapezius Muscle Exercise

Trapezius

The trapezius muscles, commonly known as the traps, are situated at the upper and middle portion of the back. They are divided into three sections – upper, middle and lower – with each having its own corresponding function:

- *upper trap:* elevates the lateral aspect of the scapula

- *middle trap:* adducts the scapula, moving it closer to the spine

- *lower trap:* depresses the scapula, maintaining it against the ribs.

Figure 13.2 Trapezius muscle

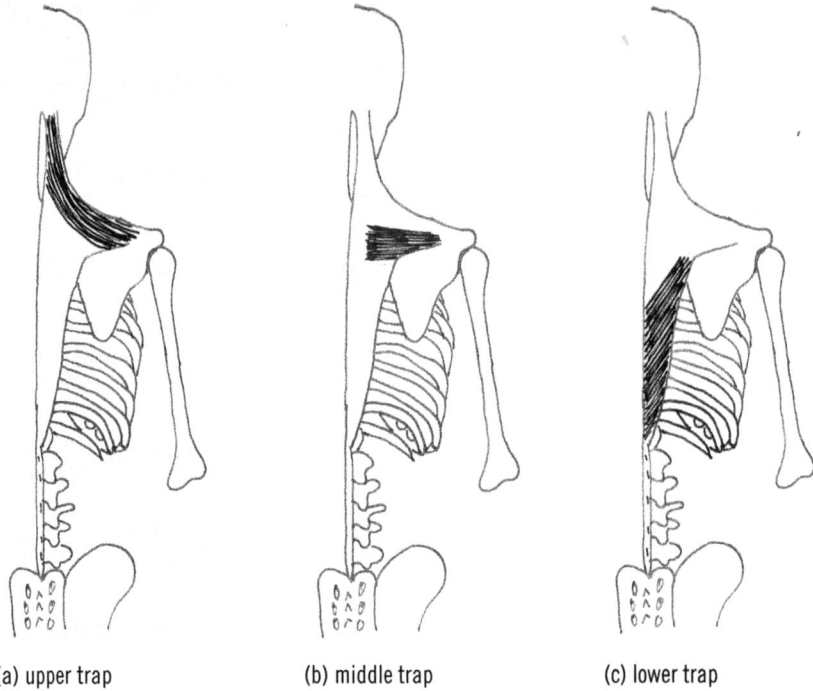

(a) upper trap (b) middle trap (c) lower trap

ORIGIN ATTACHMENT	INSERTION ATTACHMENT
• **Skull** (external occipital protuberance) • **Ligamentum nuchae** • **Spinous processes** (C7 – T12) • **Supraspinal ligament** (C7 – T12)	• **Scapula** (both the acromion process and the full length of scapula spine)

Things to consider:

☑ Leaning slightly forward during a dumbbell shrug, increases leverage and range of motion.

☑ Focus during the exercise should be on raising the shoulder toward the ear.

DUMBBELL SHRUG

Standing: Superior Trapezius

Start:

Adopt a unilateral stance (see page 47 for an explanation). Securing the opposing hand to a stable structure, bend the upper body slightly forward, rotate the arm at the shoulder, grabbing the dumbbell with the working hand in a semi-supine position.

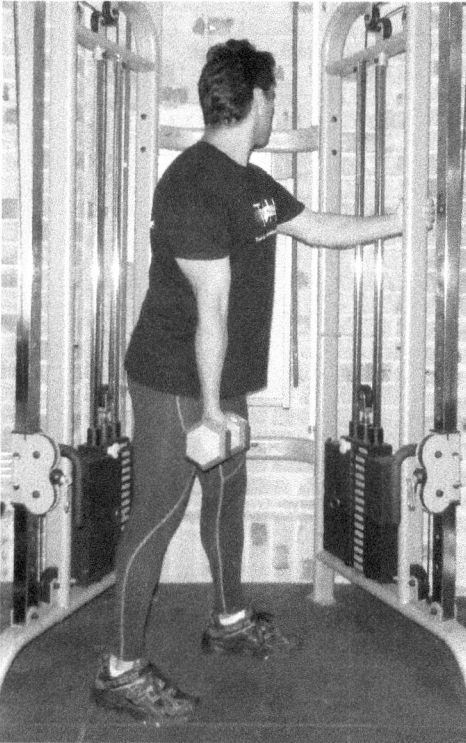

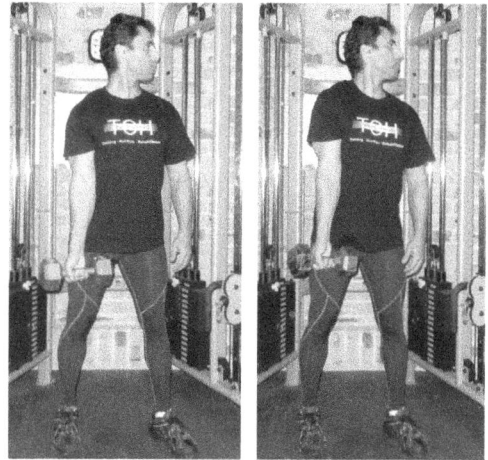

Front view

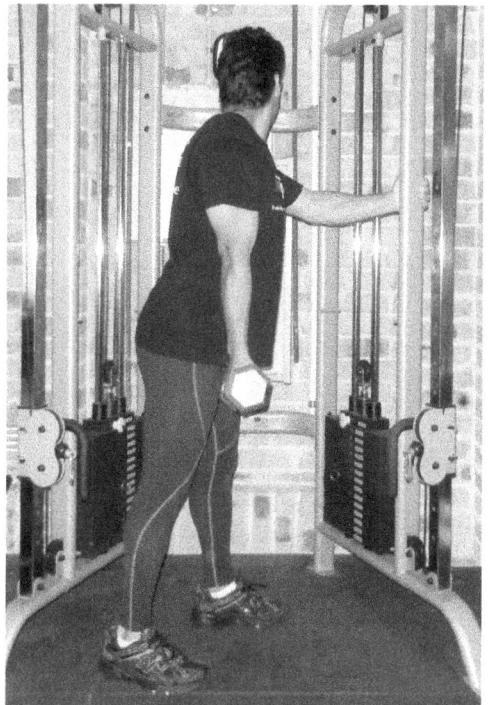

Finish:

Raise the working arm moving the shoulder toward the ear in a medial direction.

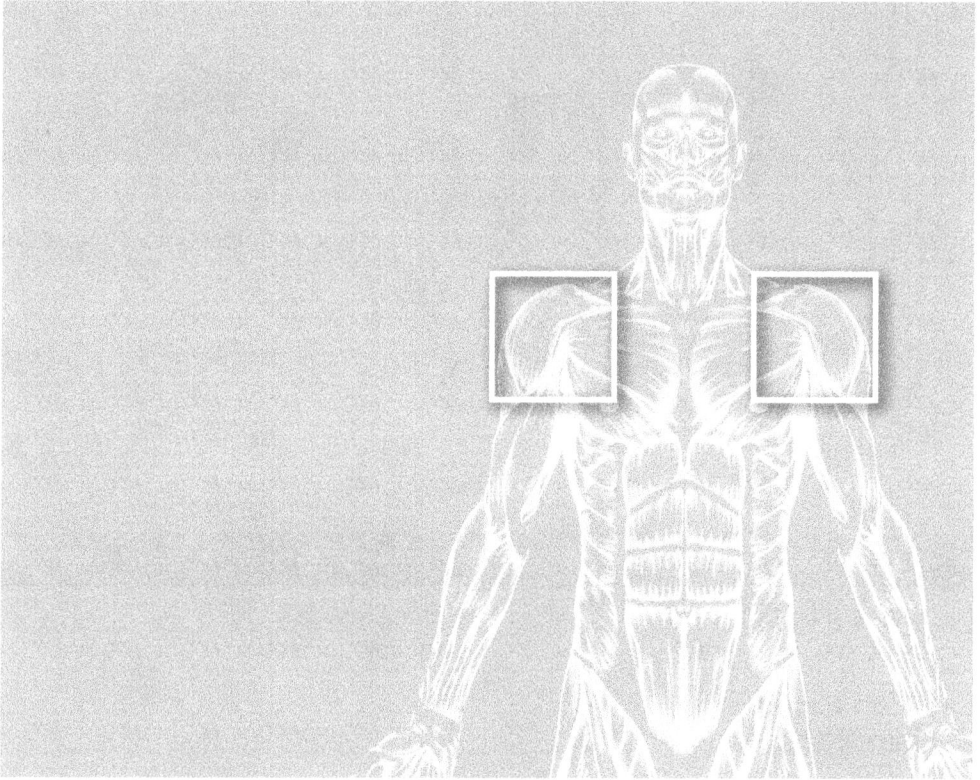

Deltoid Muscle Exercises

Deltoideus

The deltoideus muscles, commonly known as the deltoids or delts, are what most people refer to as the shoulder muscles.

The deltoid is a muscle with three different portions: anterior, middle and posterior with each having its own function:

- *anterior deltoid:* flexes and inwardly rotates the arm
- *middle deltoid:* abducts the arm
- *posterior deltoid:* extends and outwardly rotates the arm.

Figure. 13.3 Deltoideus muscle

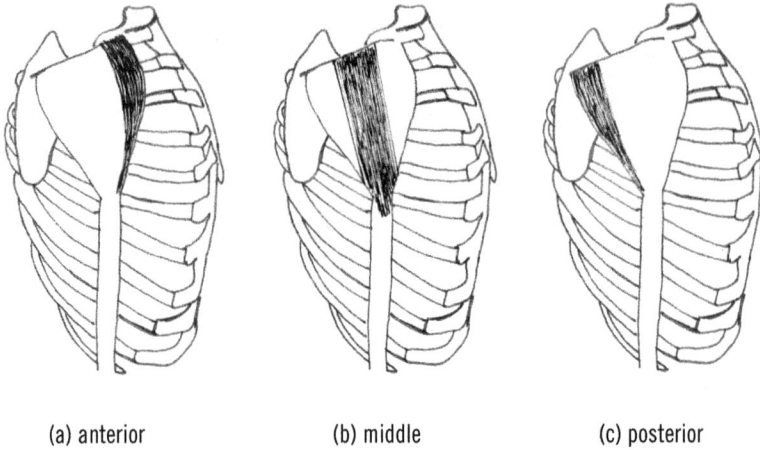

(a) anterior (b) middle (c) posterior

ORIGIN ATTACHMENT	INSERTION ATTACHMENT
• **Anterior – clavicle** (front, top, lateral end) • **Middle – scapula** (acromion process) • **Posterior – scapula** (lateral end of scapula spine)	• **Humerus** (deltoid tuberosity)

Things to consider:

☑ Developing all three portions of each deltoid muscle is important for aesthetic purposes, injury prevention and stabilisation of the shoulder region.

☑ The posterior portion of the deltoid helps to prevent forward displacement of the head of the humerus.

☑ Shoulder width is created by the middle portion.

☑ Range of movement of the arm across the body created by the anterior portion of the deltoid will be restricted due to the position of ligaments and the shoulder capsule being connected firmly at the top.

☑ Restrict elbow joint movement during anterior deltoid bent-arm exercise.

☑ Restrict elbow joint movement during posterior deltoid exercises.

☑ Hand position for deltoid muscle exercises will be created via the elbow and shoulder joints.

LATERAL DUMBBELL RAISE

Standing: Middle Deltoid – Straight Arm

Start:

Adopt a unilateral stance (see page 47 for an explanation). Secure the opposing hand to a stable structure and grab the dumbbell, placing the working hand in a neutral (thumb up) position.

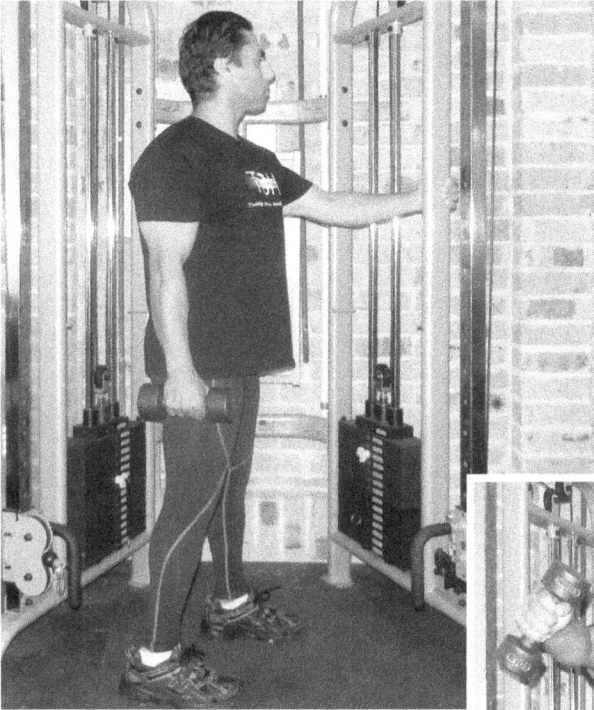

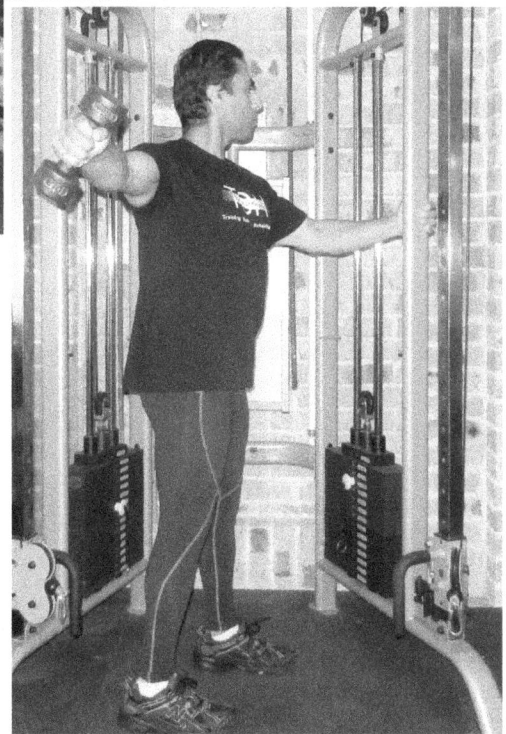

Finish:

Abduct the working arm at the shoulder joint in a lateral, backward direction to shoulder height, concluding with the hand in a semi-prone position.

Standing: Middle Deltoid – Bent Arm

Start:

Adopt a unilateral stance (see page 47 for an explanation). Secure the opposing hand to a stable structure and place the working arm at 90° at shoulder height, grabbing the dumbbell with the working hand in a semi-prone position.

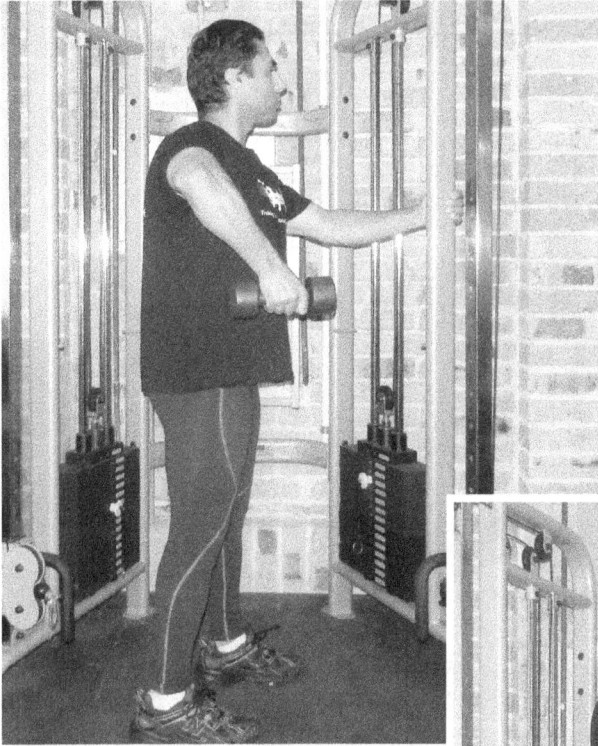

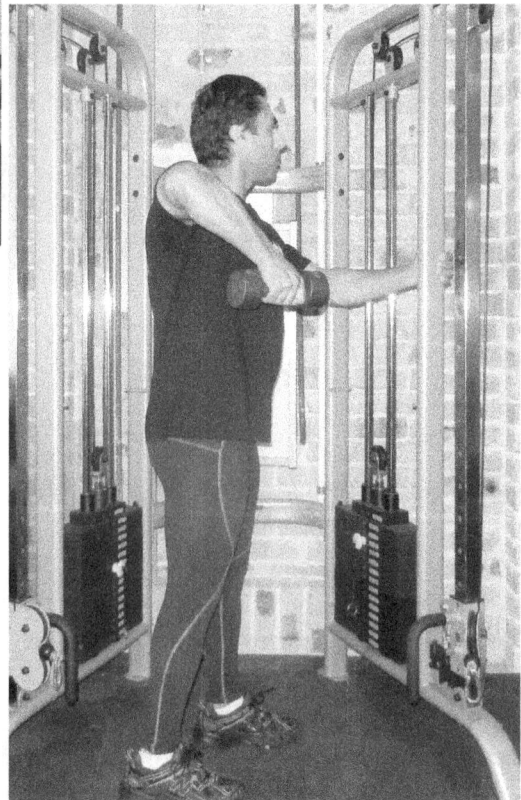

Finish:

Abduct the working arm at the shoulder joint in a lateral, backward direction above shoulder height.

ANTERIOR DUMBBELL RAISE

Standing: Anterior Deltoid – Straight Arm

Start:

Adopt a unilateral stance (see page 47 for an explanation). Secure the opposing hand to a stable structure and grab the dumbbell, placing the working hand in a semi-supine position.

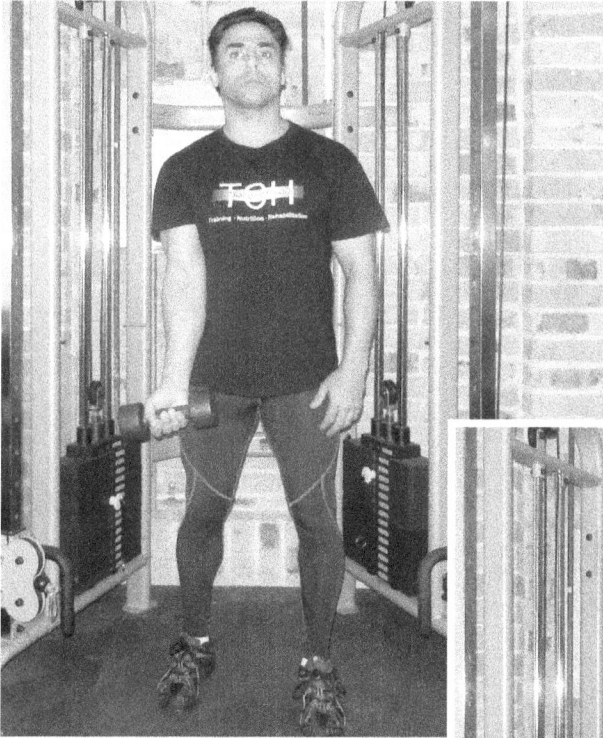

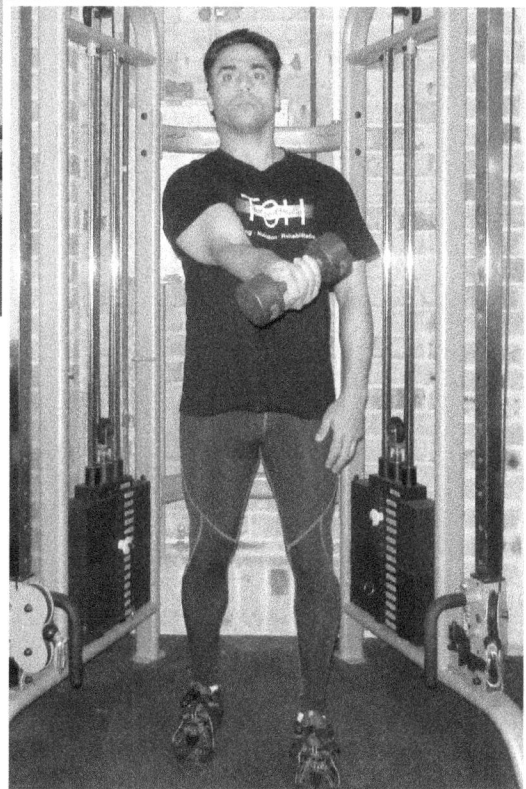

Finish:

Flex the working arm at the shoulder joint in a medial direction to lower chest height.

(*Note:* Though not evident in the photographs, the opposing hand must be secured to a stable structure.)

ANTERIOR DUMBBELL PRESS

Standing: Anterior Deltoid – Bent Arm

Start:

Adopt a unilateral stance (see page 47 for an explanation). Secure the opposing hand to a stable structure and place the working arm at 90° across the body just below shoulder height, grabbing the dumbbell with the working hand in a semi-supine position.

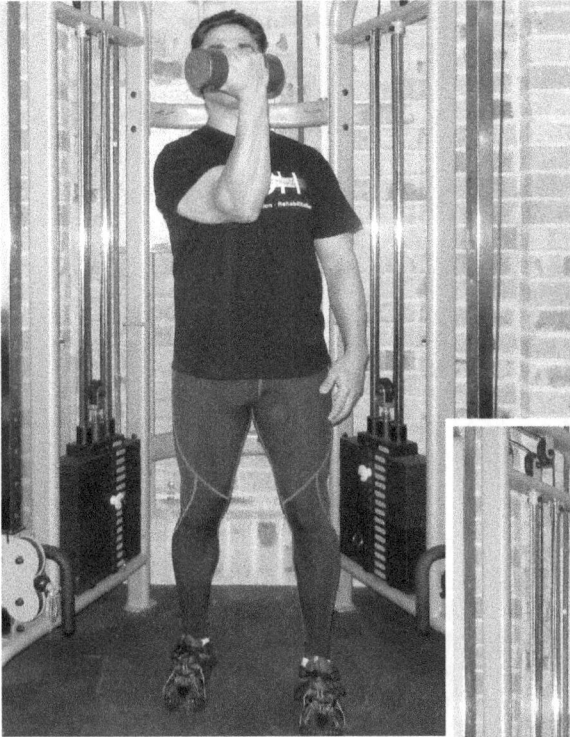

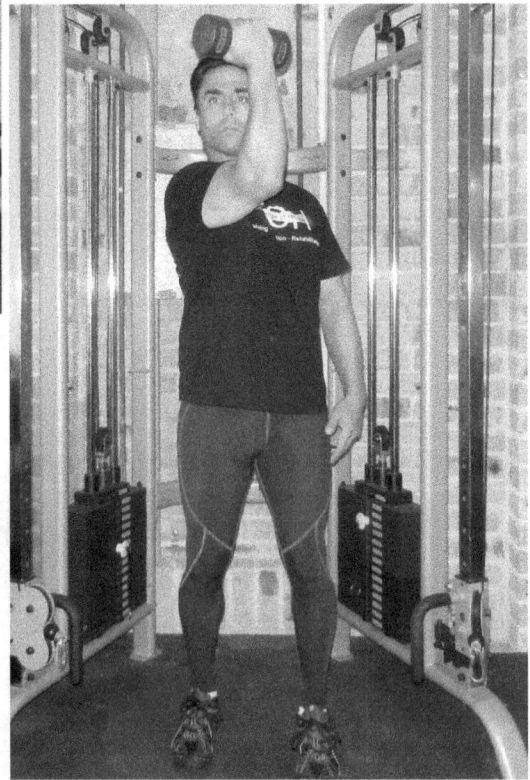

Finish:

Flex the working arm at the shoulder joint in a medial direction to shoulder height.

(*Note:* Though not evident in the photographs, the opposing hand must be secured to a stable structure.)

BENT OVER DUMBBELL RAISE

Standing: Posterior Deltoid – Straight Arm

Start:

Adopt a unilateral stance (see page 47 for an explanation) with the upper body bent over. Secure the opposing hand on the knee or a stable structure, grabbing the dumbbell with the working hand in a semi-prone position.

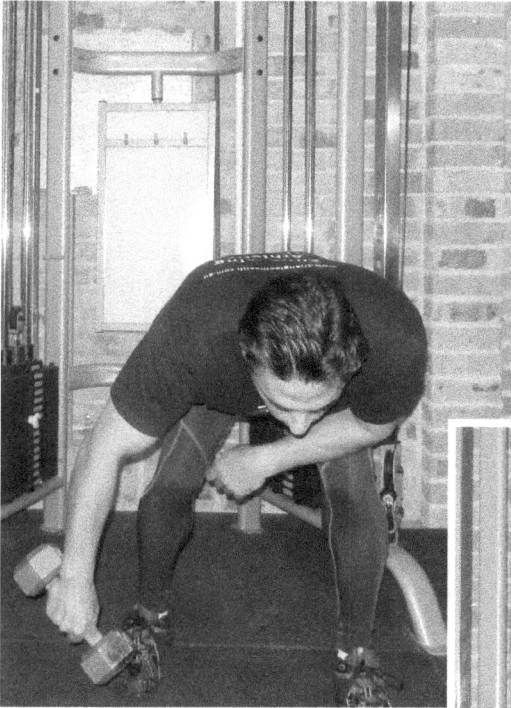

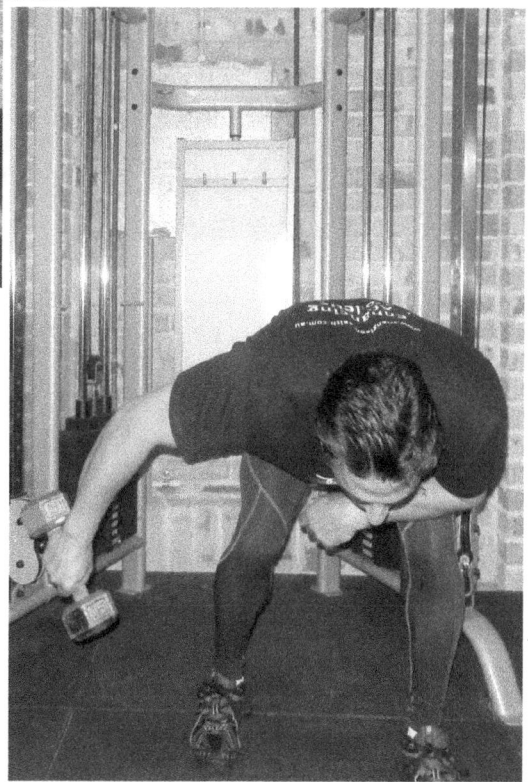

Finish:

Extend the working arm at the shoulder joint in a lateral direction below shoulder height.

(*Note:* Though not evident in the photographs, the opposing hand can alternatively be secured to a stable structure.)

Standing: Posterior Deltoid – Bent Arm

Start:

Adopt a unilateral stance (see page 47 for an explanation) with the upper body bent over. Secure the opposing hand on the knee or a stable structure, and bend the working arm 90°, grabbing the dumbbell with the working hand in a semi-prone position.

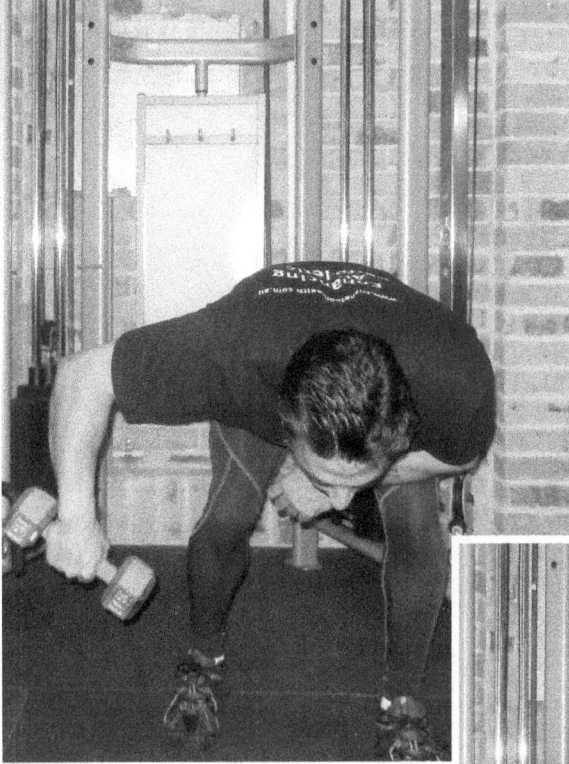

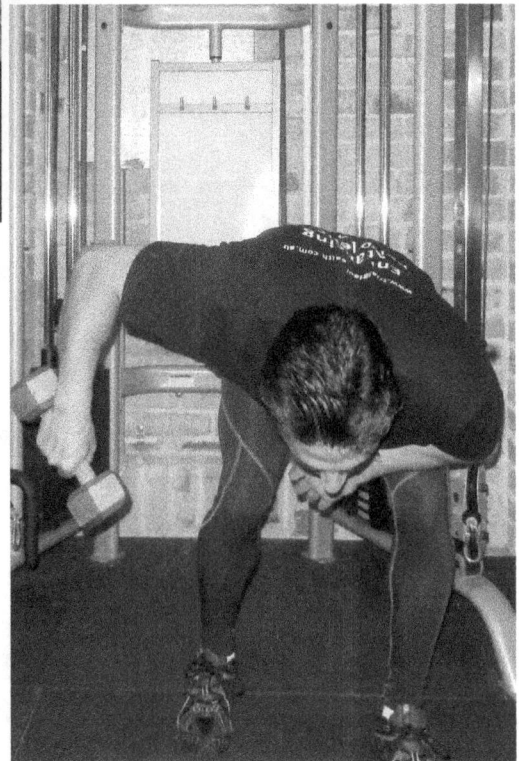

Finish:

Extend the working arm at the shoulder joint in a lateral direction so that the elbow joint is just above shoulder height.

(*Note:* Though not evident in the photographs, the opposing hand can alternatively be secured to a stable structure.)

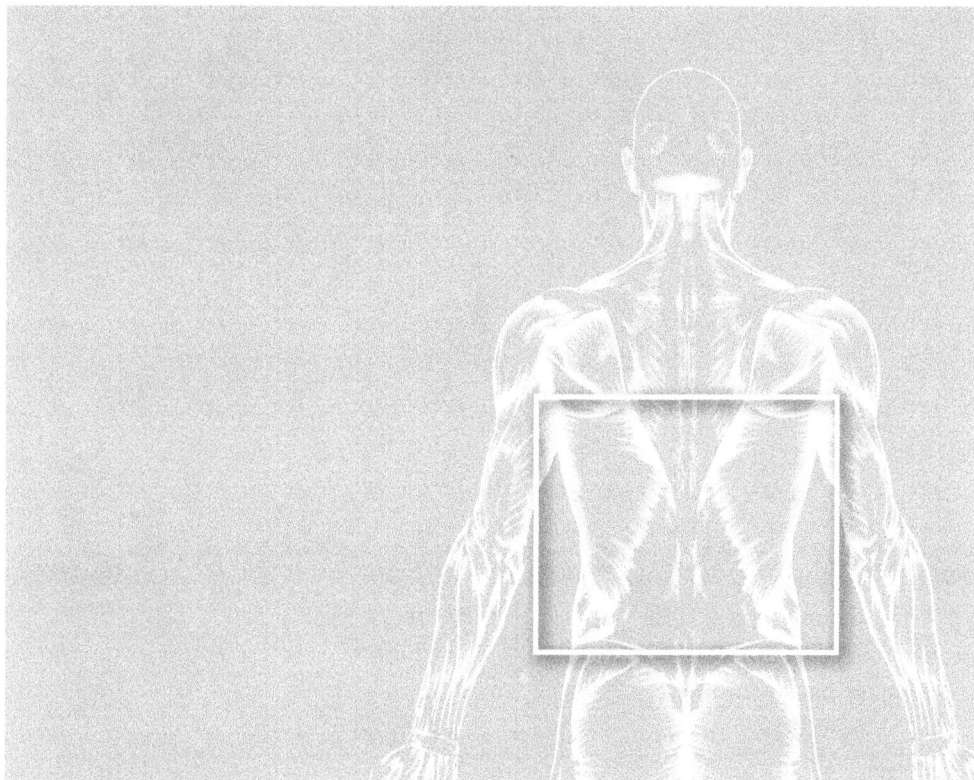

Latissimus Dorsi Muscle Exercises

Latissimus Dorsi

The latissimus dorsi muscles, or 'lats' as they are commonly called, are shoulder muscles situated to the rear of the upper body.

Similar to the fibres in the chest muscle pectoralis major, the muscle fibres at the insertion point of the lats twist 180° so that the front fibres of the tendon end up facing backward and the rear fibres end up facing forward, subsequently catering to various movements.

The latissimus dorsi muscles function to create movements of extension, adduction and medial rotation of the arm. They also maintain the bottom angle of the scapula against the rib cage.

Figure 13.4 Latissimus dorsi muscle

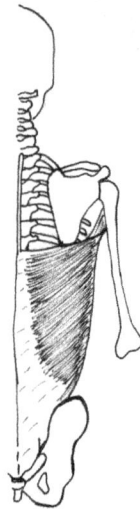

ORIGIN ATTACHMENT	INSERTION ATTACHMENT
• **T6 – sacrum** (spinous processes) • **Surpaspinal ligament** (T6 – sacrum) • **Pelvis** (illiac crest) • **Lumbar region** (fascia) • **Ribs** (bottom 3–4) • **Scapula** (bottom angle)	• **Humerus** (bicipital groove)

Things to consider:

☑ Latissimus dorsi muscles cover the middle and lower part of the back.

☑ Exercising the latissimus dorsi muscle in various aspects caters to the different fibre angles.

☑ Rotation of the body will assist in isolating various aspects of the lats.

☑ Bending knees during seated row exercises relieves pressure on the lower back.

☑ Hand position for latissimus dorsi muscle exercises will be created via the elbow and shoulder joints.

CABLE-PULLEY LAT PULLDOWN

Seated: Inferior – Lateral Aspect

Start:

Place the whole body on the same side of the working arm and rotate towards it. Secure the opposing hand and leg over and under a fixed part of a structure (such as a pad). With the working arm extended, grab the stirrup handle with the working hand in a semi-supine position.

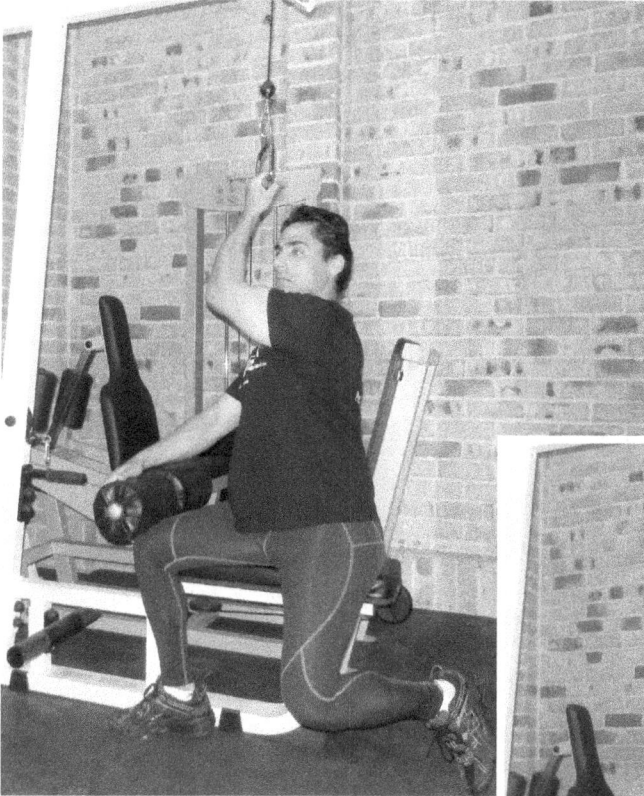

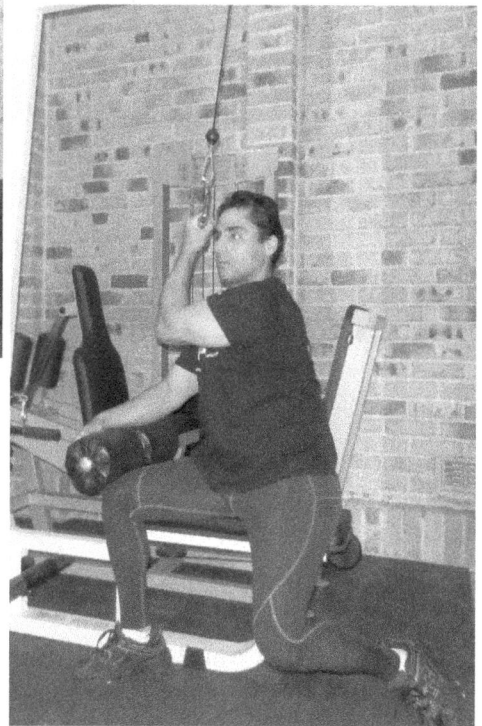

Finish:

Extend the working arm at the shoulder joint in a medial direction, reaching below shoulder height.

Seated: Superior– Lateral Aspect

Start:

Place the whole body on the opposite side of the working arm and rotate away from it. Secure the opposing hand and leg over and under a fixed part of a structure (such as a pad). With the arm at 90°, grab the stirrup handle with the working hand in a semi-supine position.

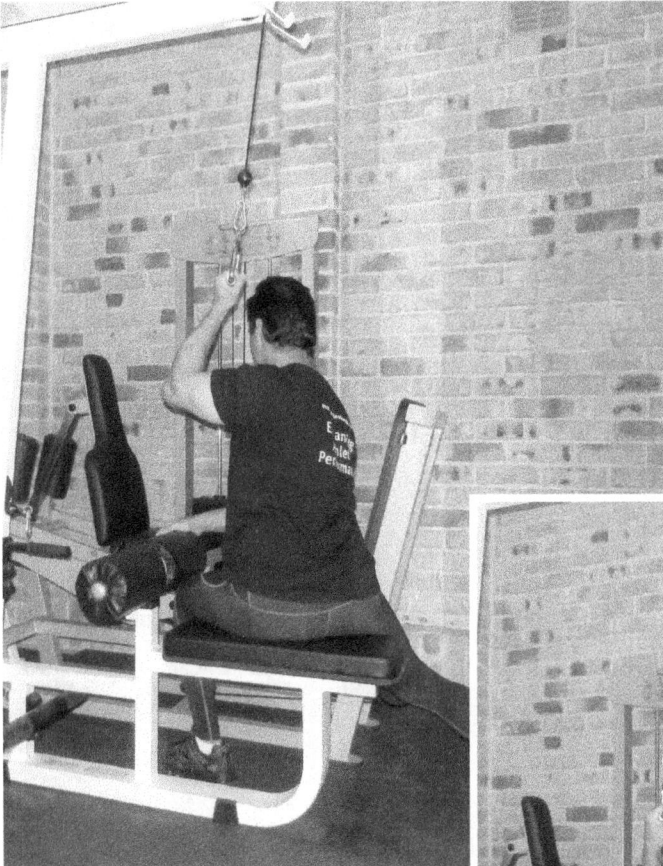

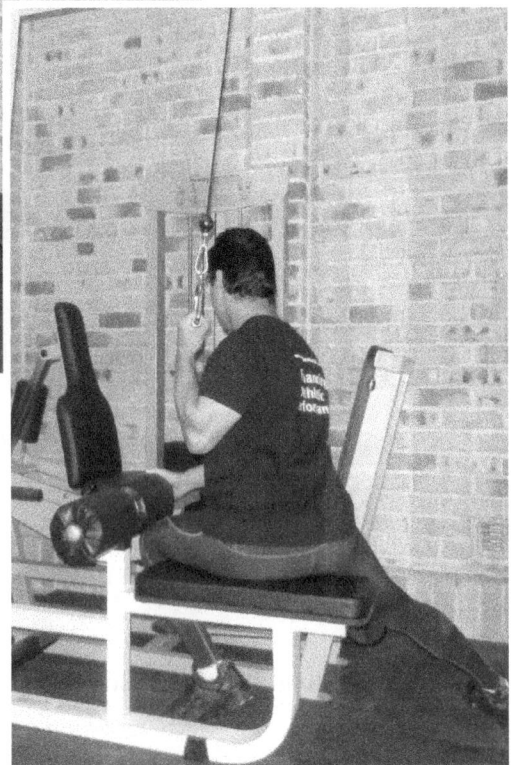

Finish:

Extend the working arm at the shoulder joint in a lateral direction, reaching full extension of the arm.

CABLE-PULLEY ROW

Seated: Superior – Middle/Lateral Aspect

Start:

Place the whole body on the opposite side of the working arm and rotate away from it. Secure the opposing hand and place the corresponding foot of working arm on the foot rest. With the working arm slightly bent, grab the stirrup handle with the working hand in a semi-prone position.

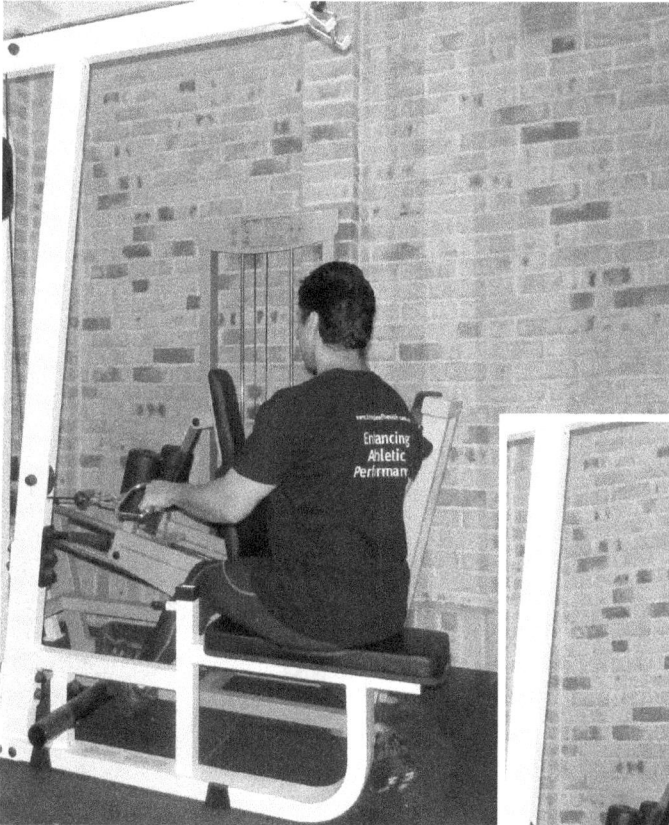

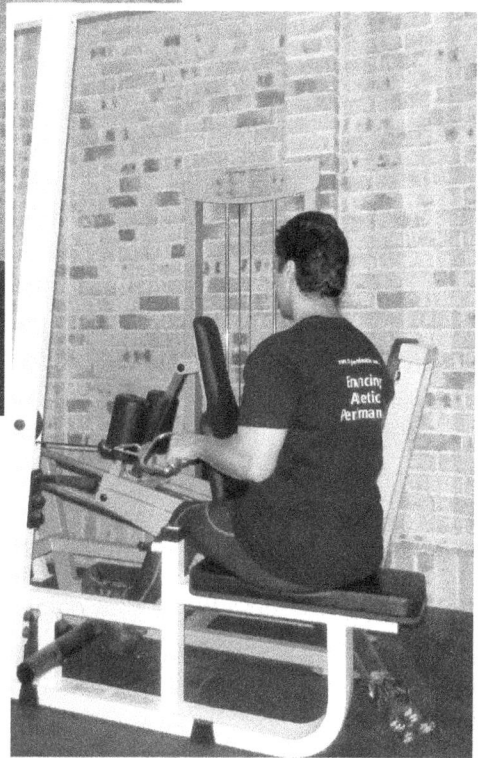

Finish:

Extend the working arm at the shoulder joint in a lateral direction, reaching 90° at the shoulder.

(*Note:* Though not evident in the photographs, the opposing hand must be secured to a stable structure.)

Seated: Superior – Middle/Medial Aspect

Start:

Place the whole body on the opposite side of the working arm and rotate away from it. Secure the opposing hand and place the corresponding foot of the working arm on the foot rest. Place the working arm at 90° at the shoulder, in a diagonal direction, and grab the stirrup handle with the working hand in a semi-prone position.

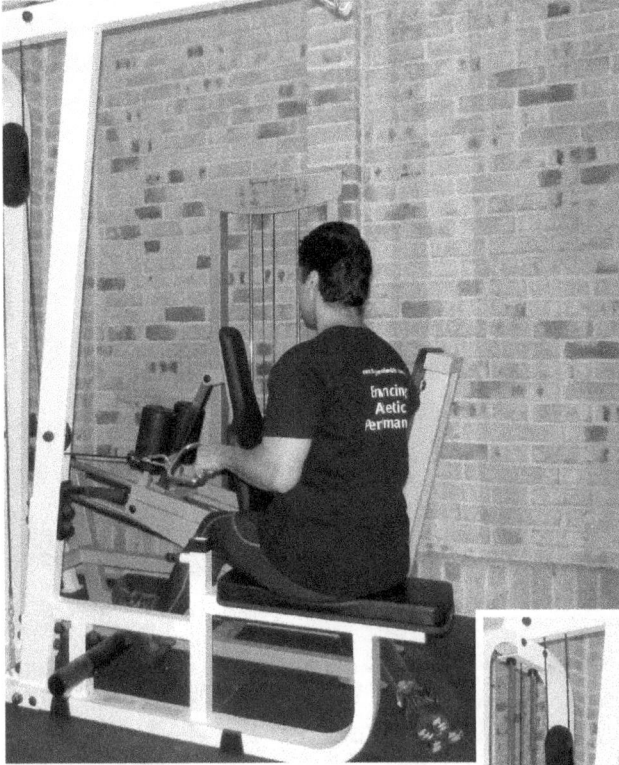

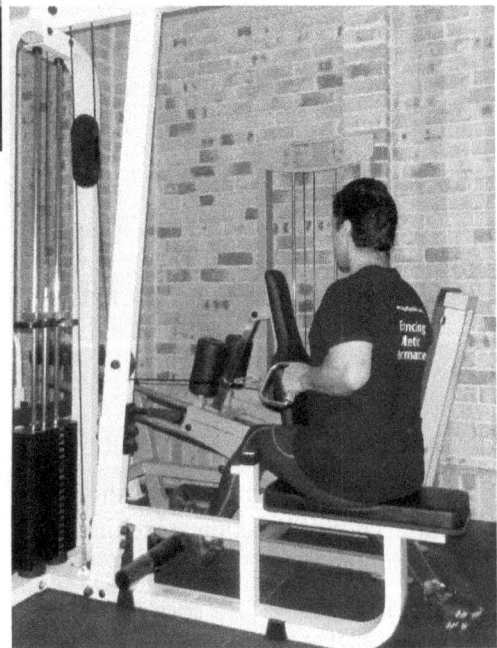

Finish:

Extend the working arm at the shoulder joint in a lateral direction to the point where the hand is in line with the waist.

(*Note:* Though not evident in the photographs, the opposing hand must be secured to a stable structure.)

Seated: Middle – Inferior/Lateral Aspect

Start:

Place the whole body on the opposite side of the working arm and rotate away from it. Secure the opposing hand and place the corresponding foot of the working arm on the foot rest. With the working arm slightly bent, grab the stirrup handle with the working hand in a semi-supine position.

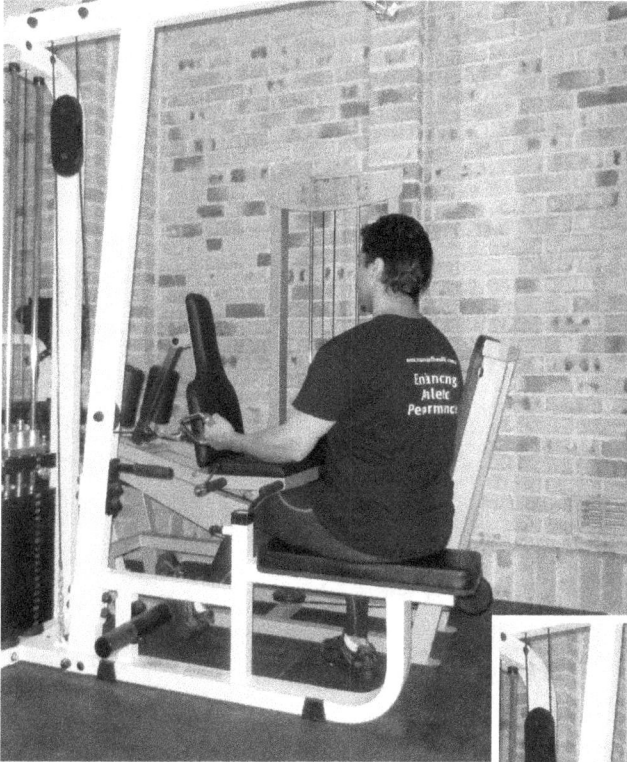

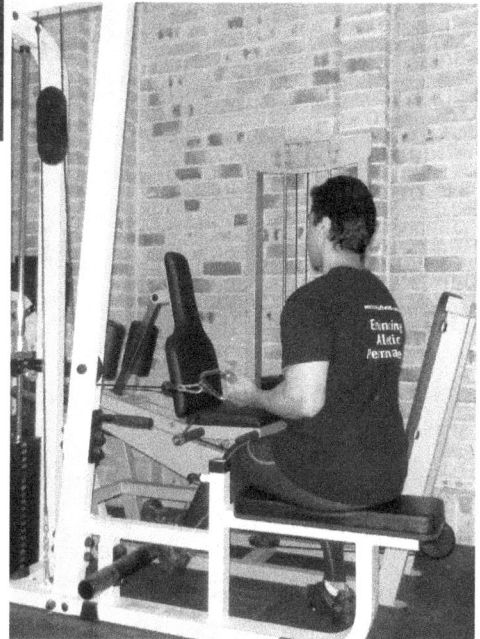

Finish:

Extend the working arm at the shoulder joint in a lateral direction, reaching 90° at the shoulder.

(*Note:* Though not evident in the photographs, the opposing hand must be secured to a stable structure.)

Seated: Middle – Inferior/Medial Aspect

Start:

Place the whole body on the opposite side of the working arm and rotate away from it. Secure the opposing hand and place the corresponding foot of the working arm on the foot rest. Place the working arm at 90° at the shoulder in a diagonal direction, and grab the stirrup handle with the working hand in a semi-supine position.

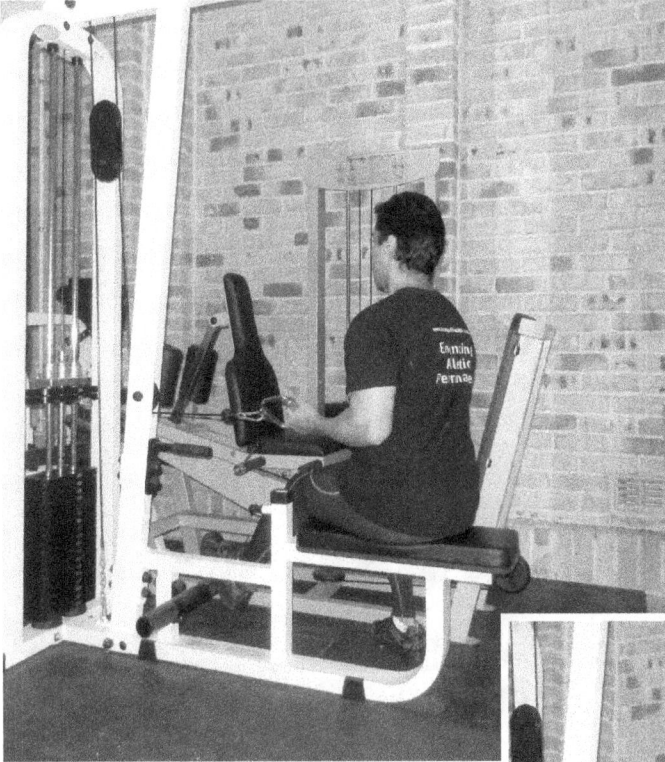

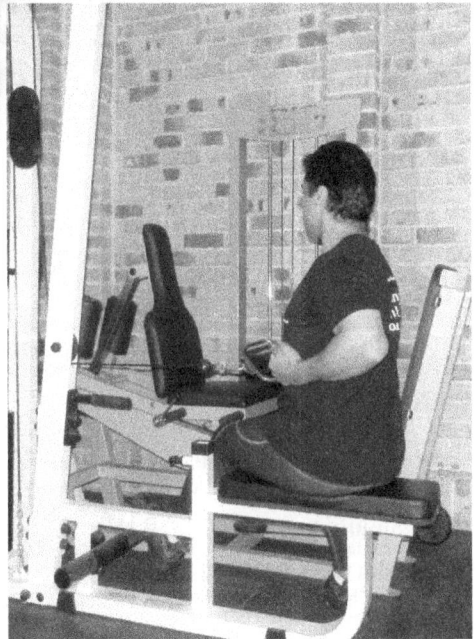

Finish:

Extend the working arm at the shoulder joint in a lateral direction to the point where the hand is in line with the waist.

(*Note:* Though not evident in the photographs, the opposing hand must be secured to a stable structure.)

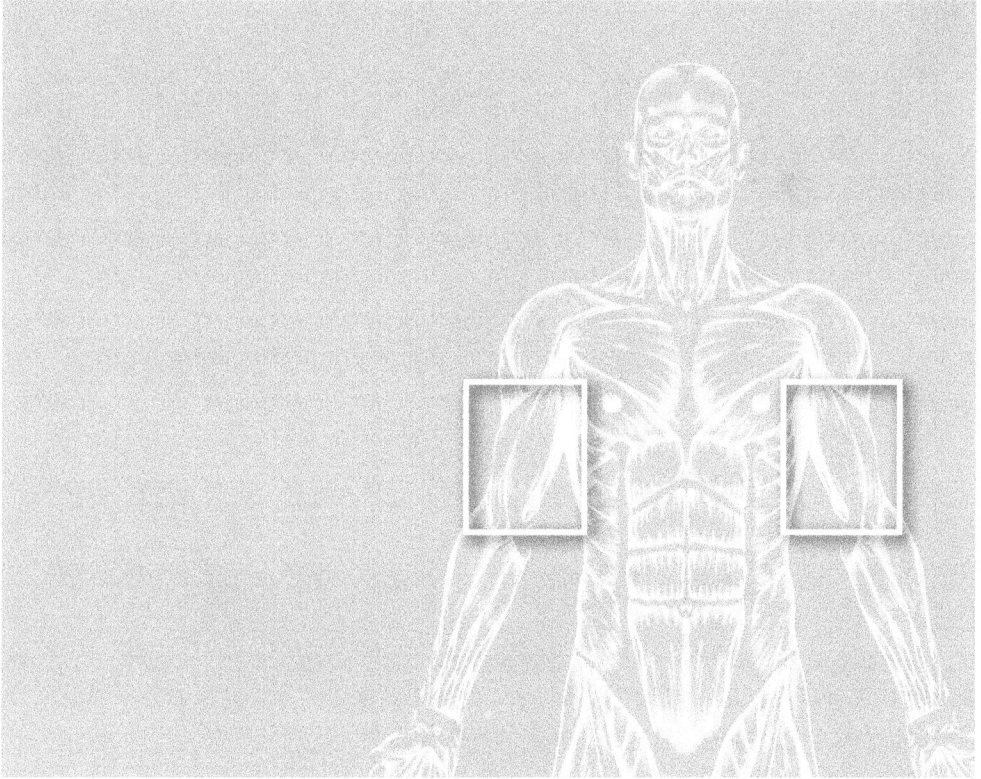

Biceps Muscle Exercises

Biceps Brachii

Most people automatically think of the biceps muscles when the arms are mentioned.

In fact, an individual arm encompasses upper and lower sections, with each section made up of multiple muscle groups that carry out various functions. This makes it imperative to develop each section and muscle group equally.

Generally, it is the triceps muscles that give the upper arm its girth but individuals differ: the arms of some people are dominated by the biceps muscles.

The biceps muscles are made up of two heads, long and short, creating separate origin attachment points and functions to create flexion of the forearm at the elbow joint, supination of the hand (due to its attachment at the radius bone) and weak flexing of the arm at the shoulder joint.

Figure 13.5 Biceps brachii muscle

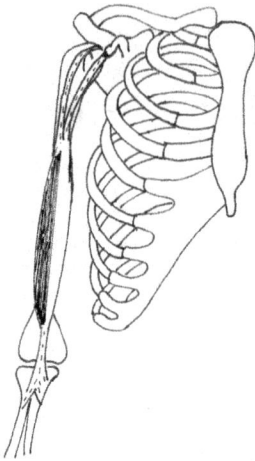

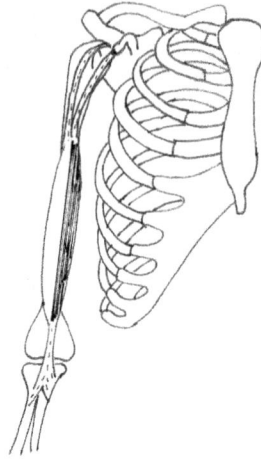

(a) long head   (b) short head

ORIGIN ATTACHMENT	INSERTION ATTACHMENT
• **Long head – scapula** (supraglenoid tubercle) • **Short head – scapula** (coracoid process)	• **Radius** (radial tuberosity, bicipital aponeurosis) • **Ulna** (fascia, medial)

Things to consider:

☑ The biceps long and short heads, lateral and medial in position, require varied positions for optimal contraction during exercise.

☑ Activation of the biceps long head is best achieved with the upper arm in an extended position.

☑ Activation of the biceps short head is best achieved with the upper arm in a flexed position.

☑ Hand position for biceps muscle exercises will be created via the elbow and shoulder joints.

DUMBBELL CURL

Standing: Inferior – Medial Aspect

Start:

Adopt a unilateral stance (see page 47 for an explanation). Secure the opposing hand to a stable structure. Grab the dumbbell with the working hand in a semi-prone position.

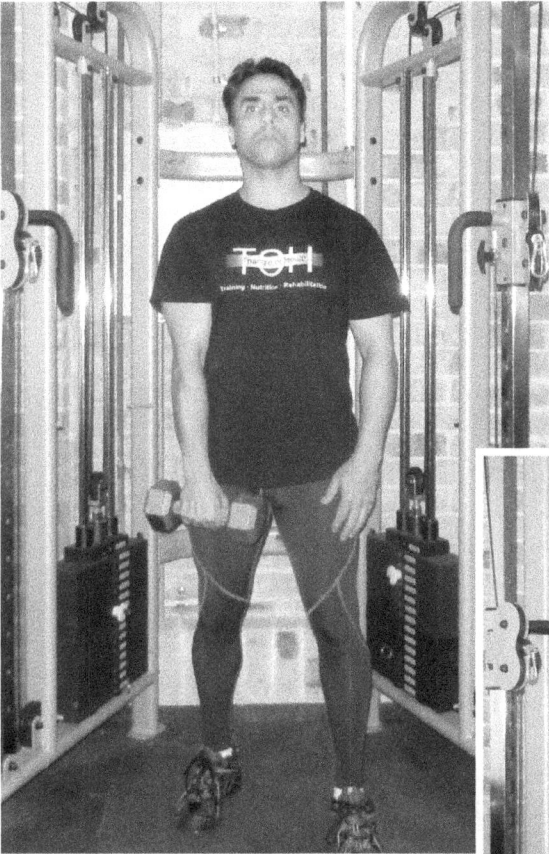

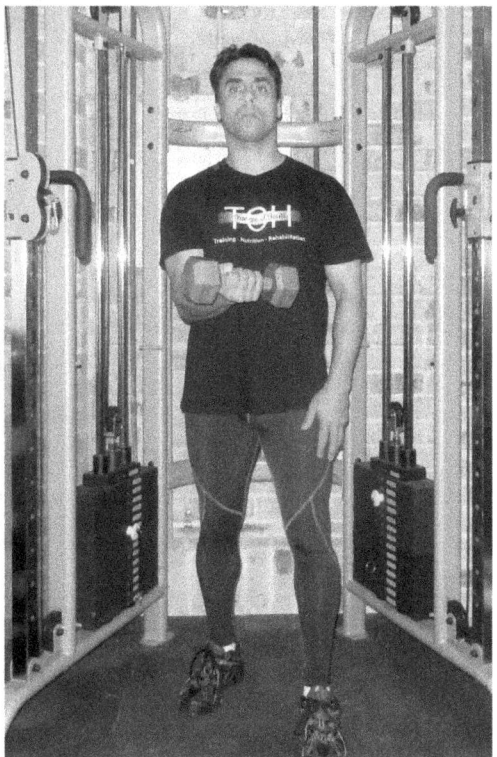

Finish:

Flex the working arm at the elbow joint in a medial direction, moving the hand into a supine position reaching 90°.

(*Note:* Though not evident in the photographs, the opposing hand must be secured to a stable structure.)

Standing: Inferior – Lateral Aspect

Start:

Adopt a unilateral stance (see page 47 for an explanation). Secure the opposing hand to a stable structure, extend and abduct the working arm at the shoulder. Grab the dumbbell with the working hand in a semi-supine position.

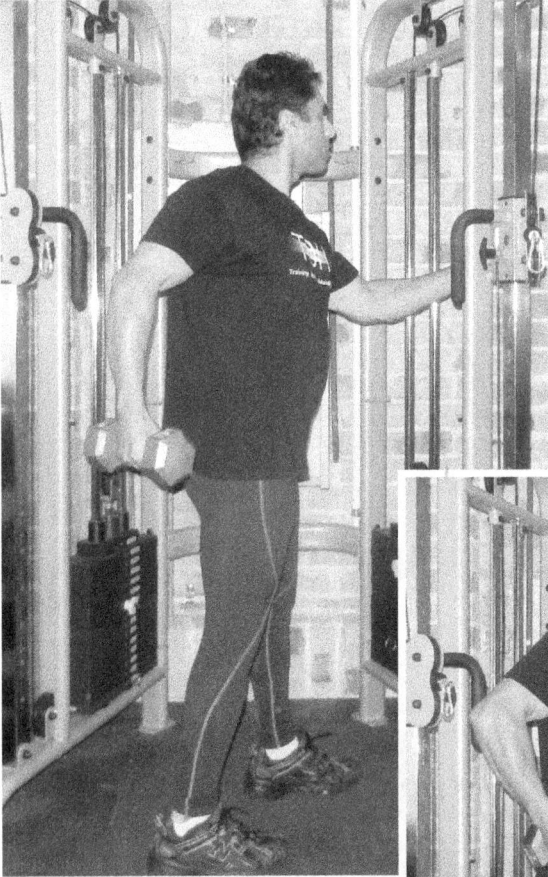

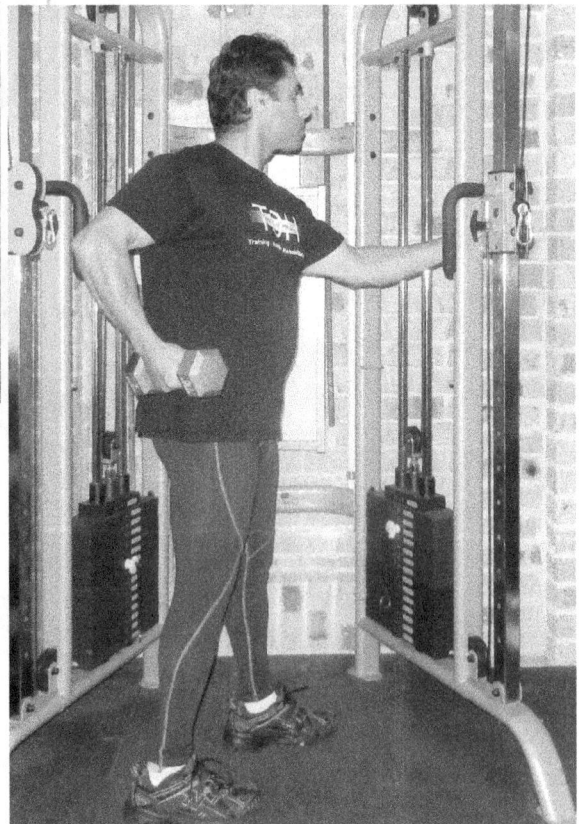

Finish:

Flex the working arm at the elbow joint in a medial direction, reaching approximately 90°.

Standing: Superior – Medial Aspect

Start:

Adopt a unilateral stance (see page 47 for an explanation). Secure the opposing hand to a stable structure and place the arm at 90° across the body, with the elbow just below shoulder height. Grab the dumbbell with the working hand in a supine position.

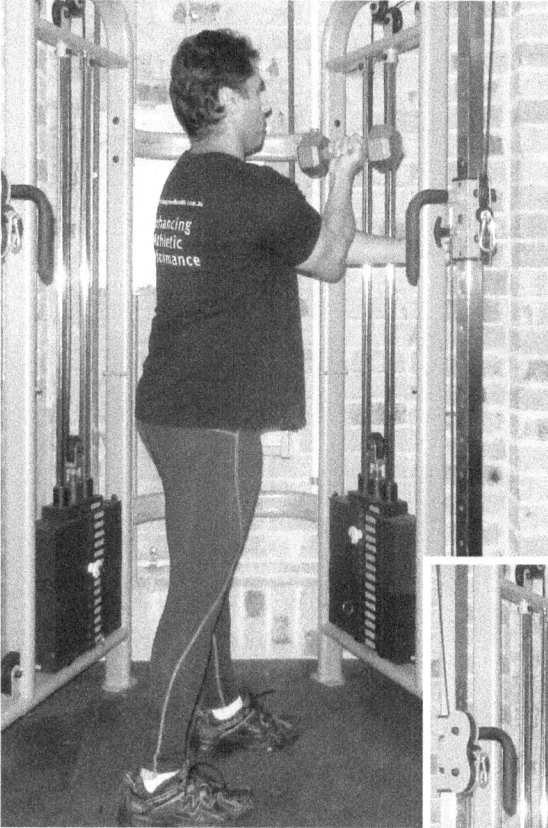

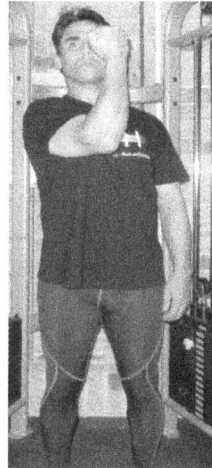

Front view

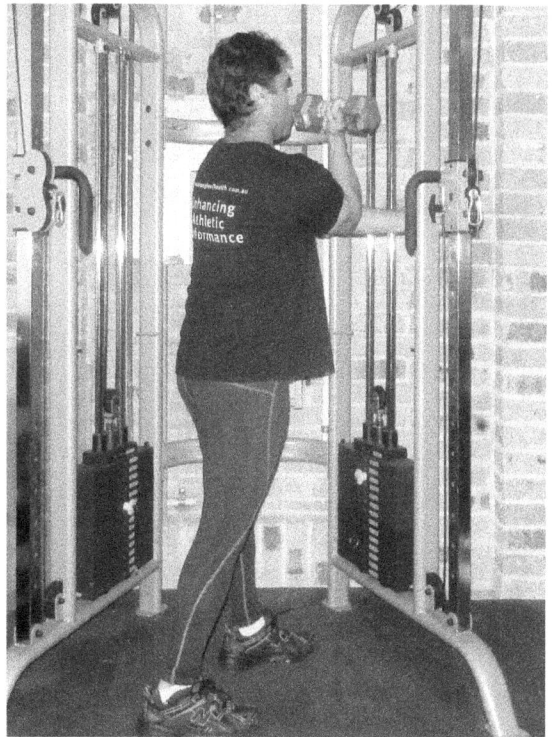

Finish:

Flex the working arm at the elbow joint in a lateral direction to the initial point where the forearm and biceps muscle touch.

Standing: Superior – Lateral Aspect

Start:

Adopt a unilateral stance (see page 47 for an explanation). Secure the opposing hand to a stable structure and place the working arm at 90° outward, with the elbow just below shoulder height. Grab the dumbbell with the working hand in a semi-supine position.

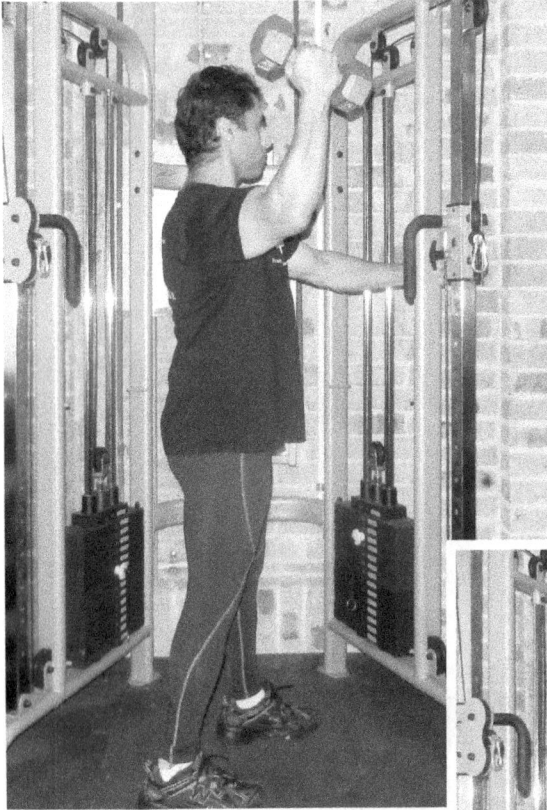

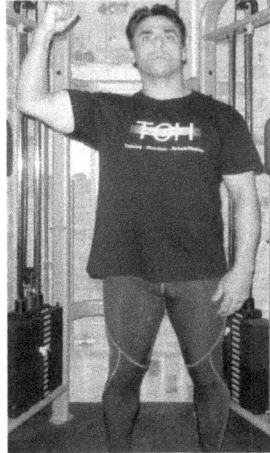

Front view

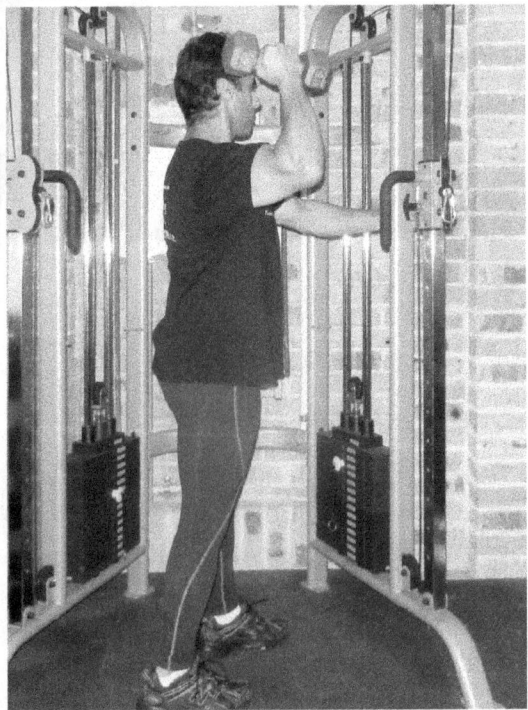

Finish:

Flex the working arm at the elbow joint in a medial direction to the initial point where the forearm and biceps muscle touch.

CABLE-PULLEY CURL

Standing: Inferior – Medial Aspect

Start:

Adopt a unilateral stance (see page 47 for an explanation). Secure the opposing hand to a stable structure. Grab the stirrup handle with the working hand in a semi-prone position.

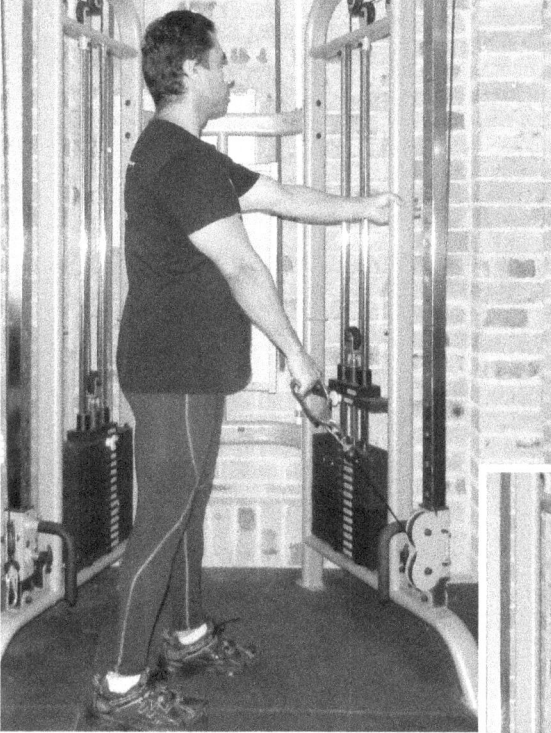

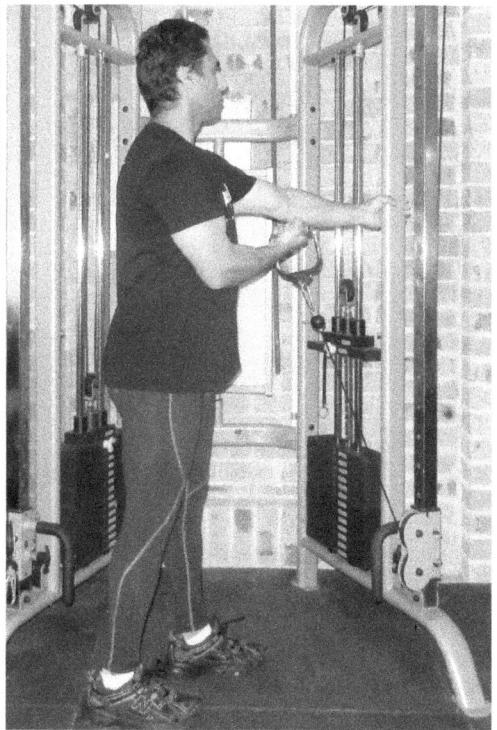

Finish:

Flex the working arm at the elbow joint in a medial direction, moving the working hand into a supine position, reaching 90° across the body.

Standing: Inferior – Lateral Aspect

Start:

Adopt a unilateral stance (see page 47 for an explanation). Secure the opposing hand to a stable structure, then extend and abduct the working arm at the shoulder. Grab the stirrup handle with the working hand in a semi-supine position.

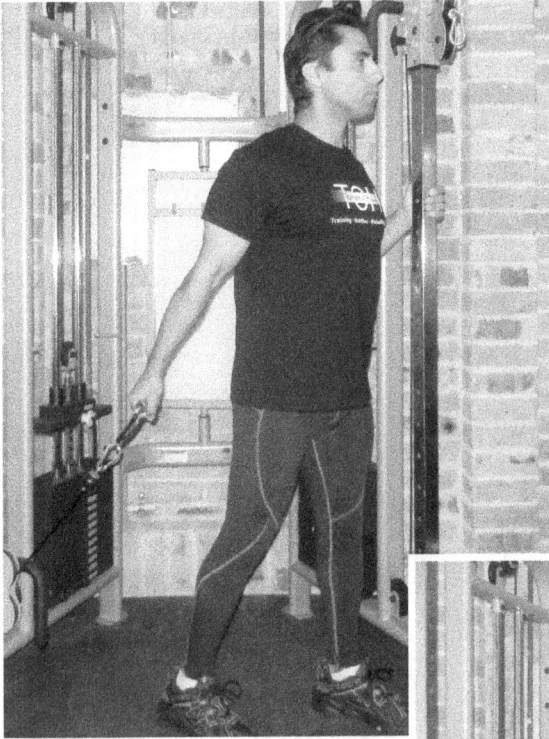

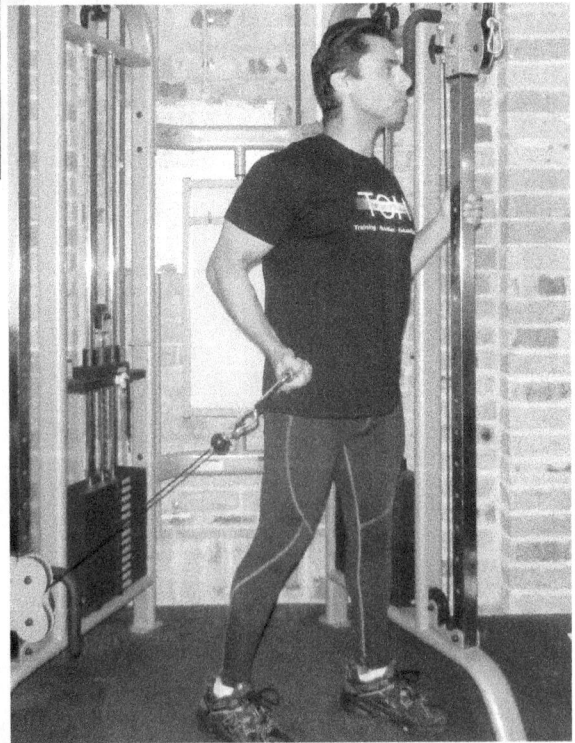

Finish:

Flex the working arm at the elbow joint in a medial direction, reaching approximately 90°.

Standing: Superior – Medial Aspect

Start:

Adopt a unilateral stance (see page 47 for an explanation). Secure the opposing hand to a stable structure and place the working arm 90° across the body, with the elbow just below shoulder height. Grab the stirrup with the working hand in a supine position.

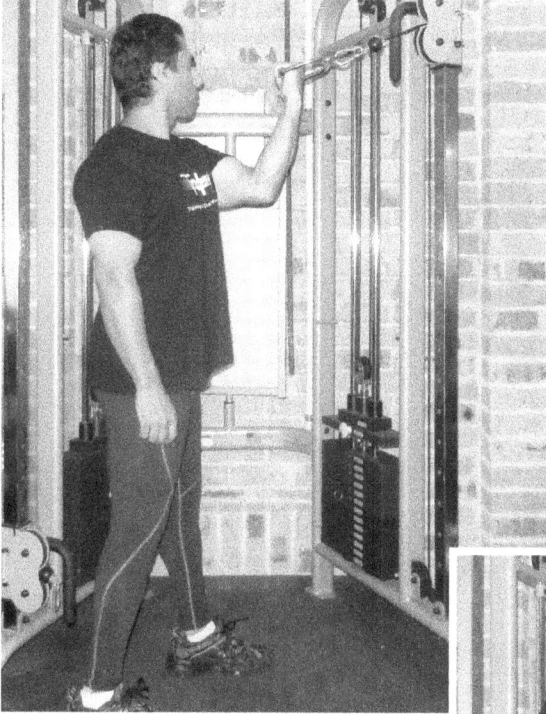

Finish:

Flex the working arm at the elbow joint in a lateral direction to the initial point where the forearm and biceps muscle touch.

(*Note:* Though not evident in the photographs, the opposing hand must be secured to a stable structure.)

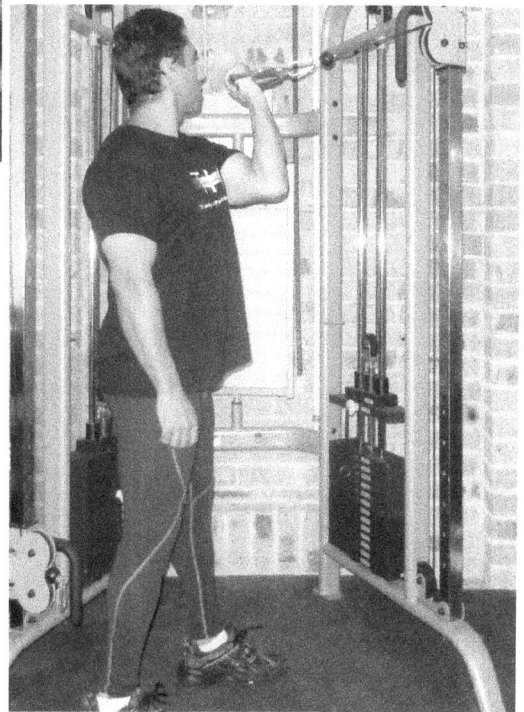

Standing: Superior – Lateral Aspect

Start:

Adopt a unilateral stance (see page 47 for an explanation). Secure the opposing hand to a stable structure and place the working arm at 90° outward, with the elbow just below shoulder height. Grab the stirrup with the working hand in a semi-supine position.

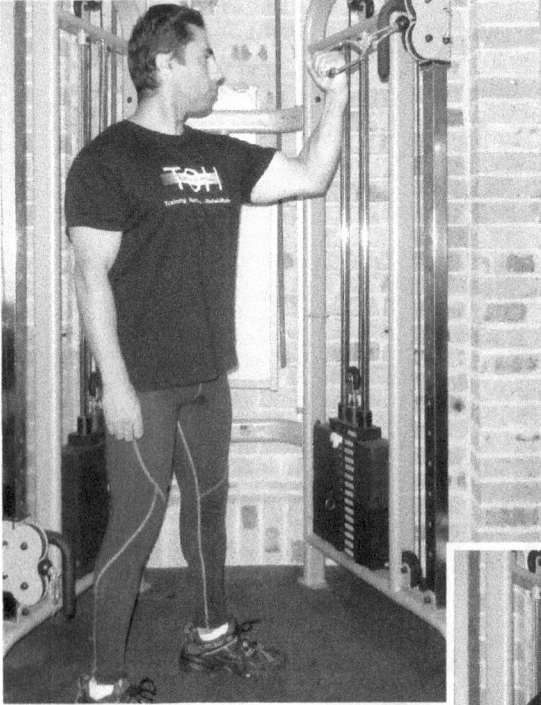

Finish:

Flex the working arm at the elbow joint in a lateral direction to the initial point where the forearm and biceps muscle touch.

(*Note:* Though not evident in the photographs, the opposing hand must be secured to a stable structure.)

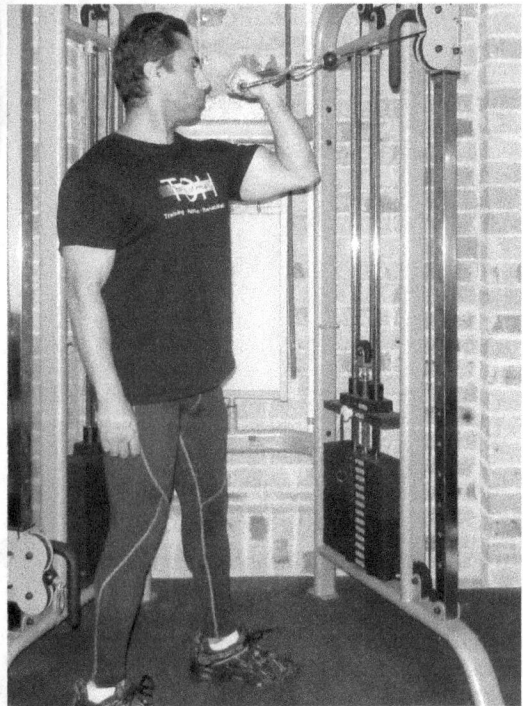

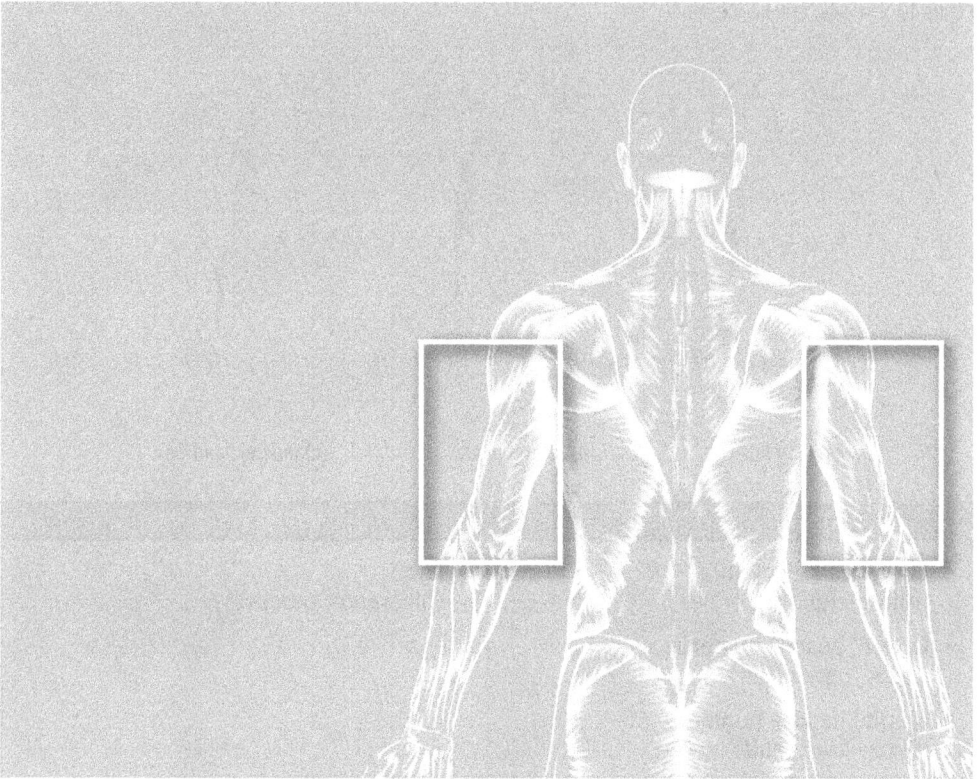

Triceps Muscle Exercises

Triceps Brachii

The majority of the upper arm is created through the triceps muscle, made up of three heads: long (largest), lateral and medial.

All three heads function to create extension of the forearm at the elbow joint, while the long head also assists in the adduction of the arm, when it is abducted at the shoulder joint.

Figure 13.6 Triceps brachii muscle

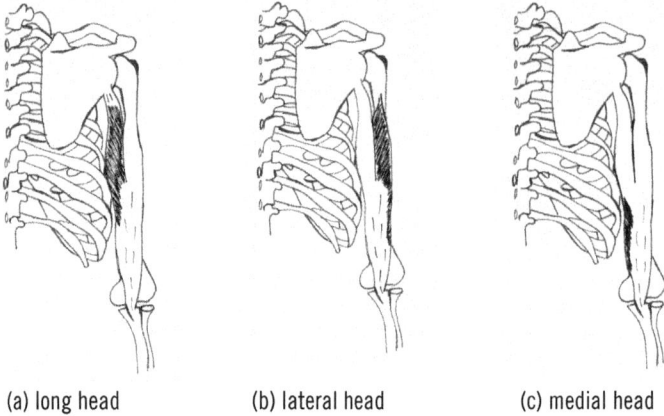

(a) long head   (b) lateral head   (c) medial head

ORIGIN ATTACHMENT	INSERTION ATTACHMENT
• **Long head – scapula** (infraglenoid tubercle) • **Lateral head – humerus** (back, upper half) • **Medial head – humerus** (back, lower half)	• **Ulna** (olecranon process)

Things to consider:

☑ Maintain alignment of the hand with the forearm so that forearm muscle recruitment is minimised during triceps contraction.

☑ All exercises must stop short of hyper-extension or locking out at the elbow joint, ensuring that jamming of the olecranon process into the fossa of the humerus – compressing the bursa sac – does not occur.

☑ Manipulating positions of the hand and arm at the elbow and shoulder joints allows isolation and lengthening of muscle heads and aspects of the triceps:

- **long head** – abduct the arm at the shoulder joint and place the hand in a semi-supine position

- **medial head** – adduct the arm at the shoulder joint and place the hand in a supine position

- **lateral head** – adduct the arm at the shoulder joint and place the hand in a neutral position

☑ Optimal contraction of the long head triceps origin attachment is best achieved via isolated movement at the shoulder joint.

DUMBBELL EXTENSION

Supine: Lateral Head

Start:

Lie supine on a flat bench. Grab the dumbbell from below with the working hand and then **use both hands to raise it**. Secure opposing hand to a stable structure, and bend working arm at 90° across the body.Grab the dumbbell with the working hand in neutral (thumb down) position.

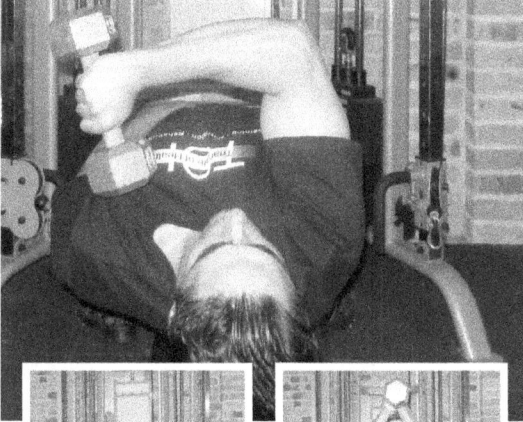

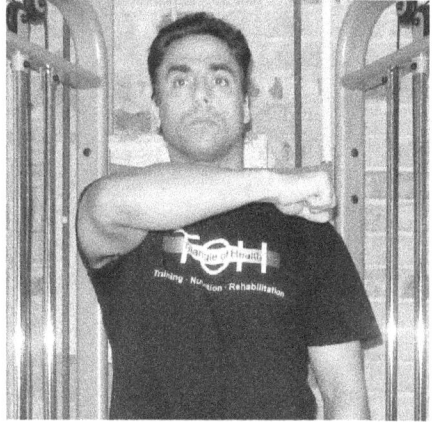

Front view

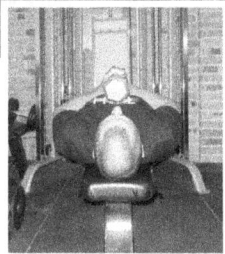

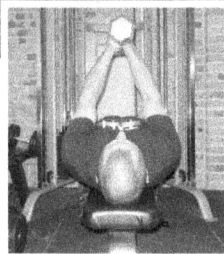

Raising dumbbell

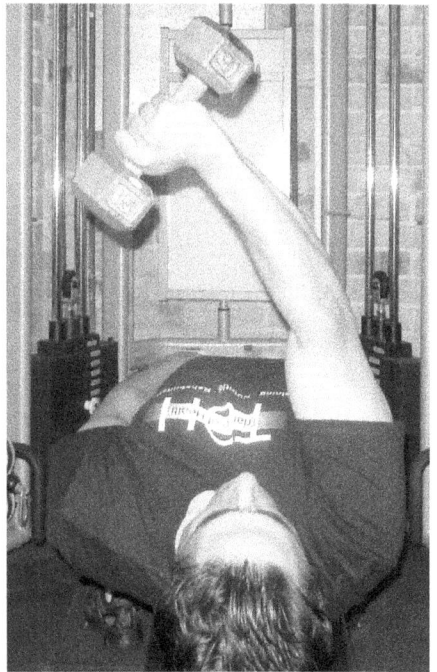

Finish:

Extend the working arm at the elbow joint, moving in a lateral direction to full extension.

(*Note:* Though not evident in the photographs, the opposing hand must be secured to a stable structure and feet placed firmly on the ground.)

Supine: Long Head – Inferior Aspect

Start:

Lie supine on a flat bench. Grab the dumbbell from below with the working hand and then **use both hands to raise it**. Secure opposing hand to a stable structure, and bend working arm at 90° and slightly abducted. Grab the dumbbell with the working hand in a semi-supine position.

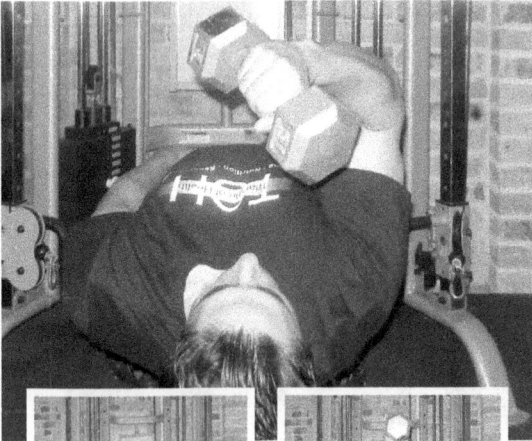

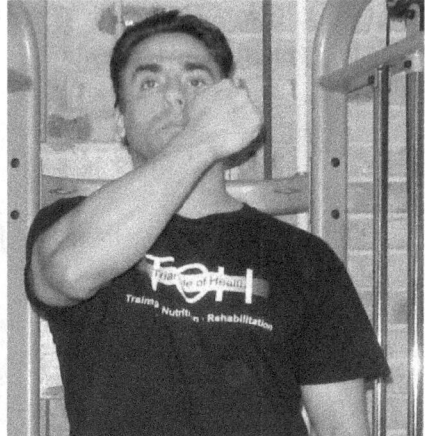

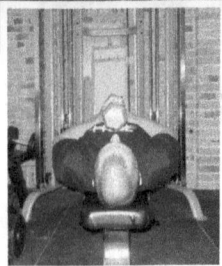

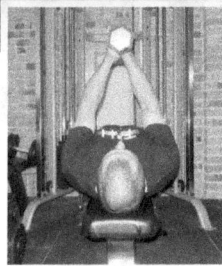

Raising dumbbell

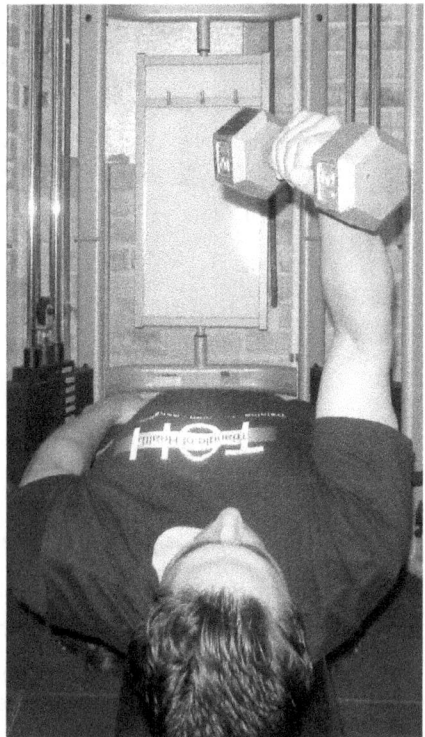

Front view

Finish:

Extend the working arm at the elbow joint, moving in a lateral direction to full extension.

(*Note:* Though not evident in the photographs, the opposing hand must be secured to a stable structure and feet placed firmly on the ground.)

Supine: Medial Head

Start:

Lie supine on a flat bench. Grab the dumbbell from below with the working hand and then **use both hands to raise it**. Secure opposing hand to a stable structure, and bend working arm at 90° adducted against the body. Grab the dumbbell with the working hand in a supine position.

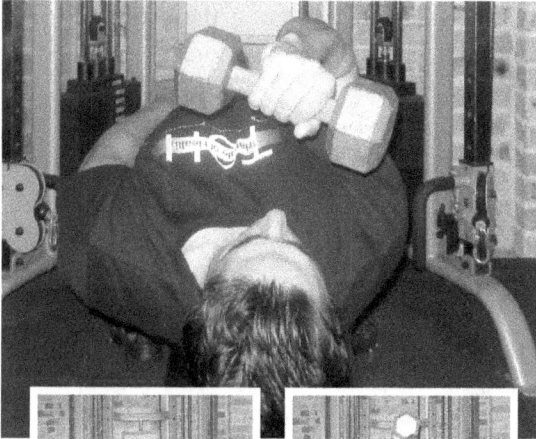

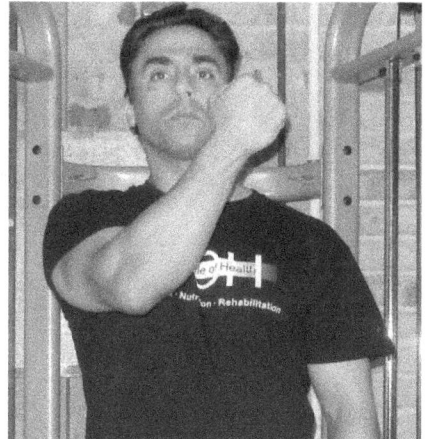

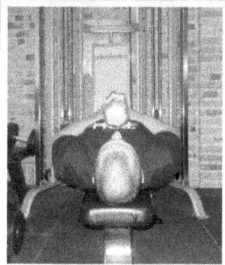

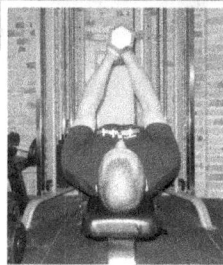

Raising dumbbell

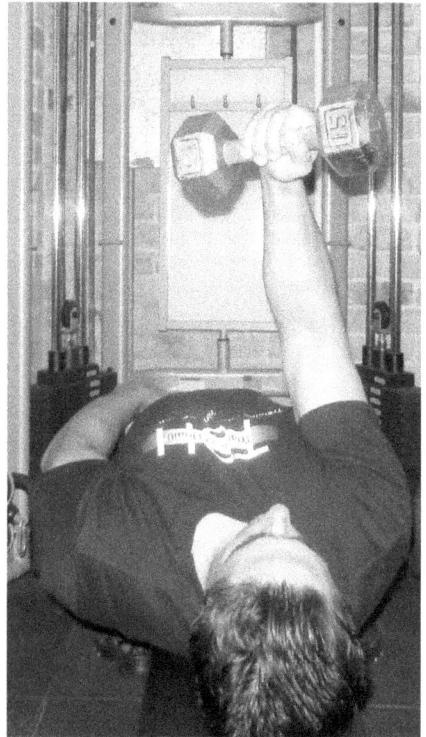

Front view

Finish:

Extend the working arm at the elbow joint, moving in a lateral direction to full extension.

(*Note:* Though not evident in the photographs, the opposing hand must be secured to a stable structure and feet placed firmly on the ground.)

DUMBBELL ADDUCTOR

Supine: Long Head – Superior Aspect

Start:

Lie supine on a flat bench. Grab the dumbbell from below with the working hand and then **use both hands to raise it**. Secure opposing hand to a stable structure, and bend working arm at elbow joint, with slight abduction at the shoulder joint. Grab the dumbbell with the working hand in a semi-supine position.

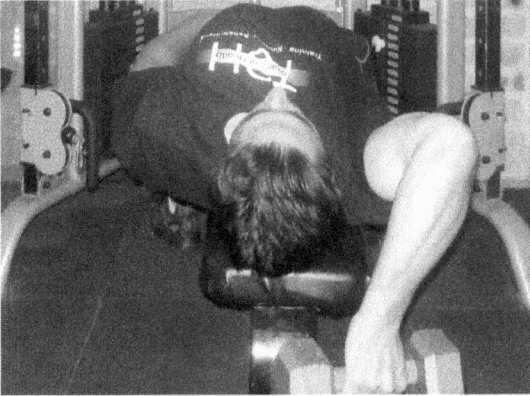

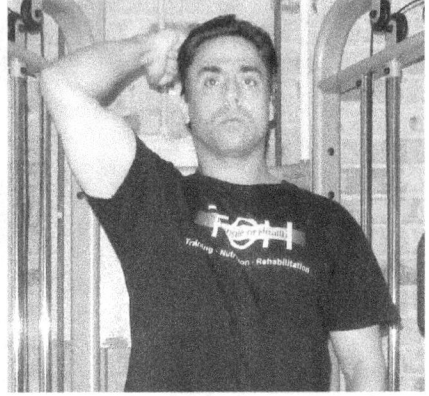

Front view

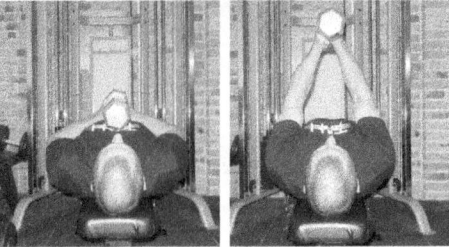

Raising dumbbell

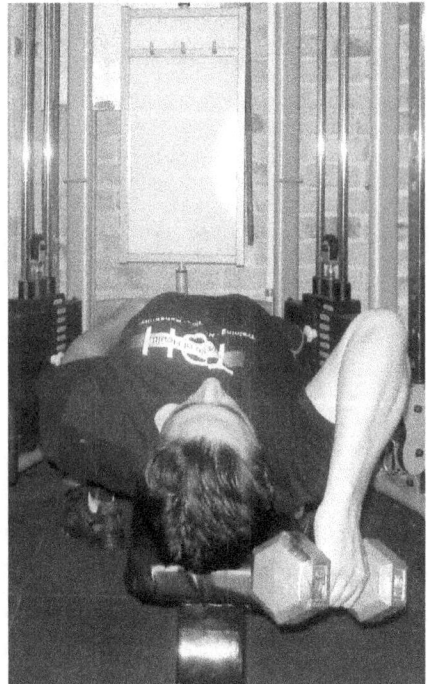

Finish:

Adduct the working arm at the shoulder joint, moving in a medial direction to the point where the elbow is pointed to the ceiling.

(*Note:* Though not evident in the photographs, the opposing hand must be secured to a stable structure and feet placed firmly on the ground.)

CABLE-PULLEY EXTENSION

Standing: Lateral Head

Start:

Adopt a unilateral stance (see page 47 for an explanation). Secure the opposing hand to a stable structure and place the working arm at 90° across the body. Grab the end of the cable with the working hand in a neutral (thumb up) position.

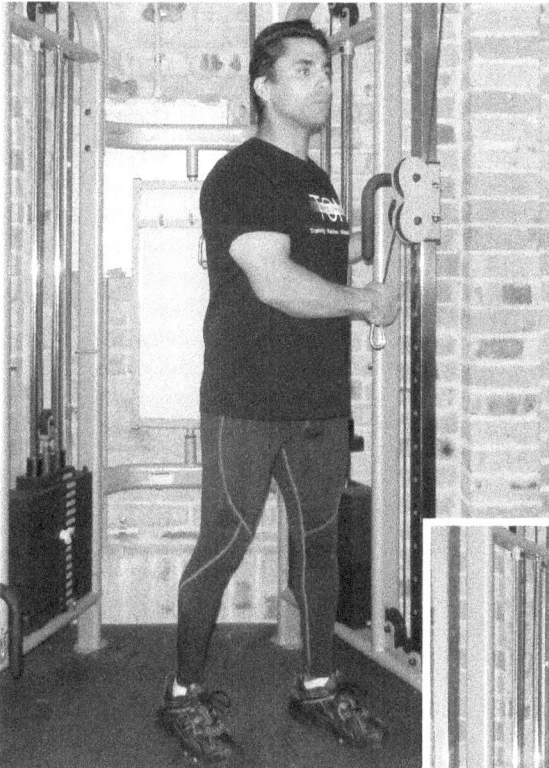

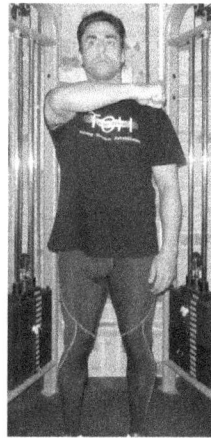

Front view

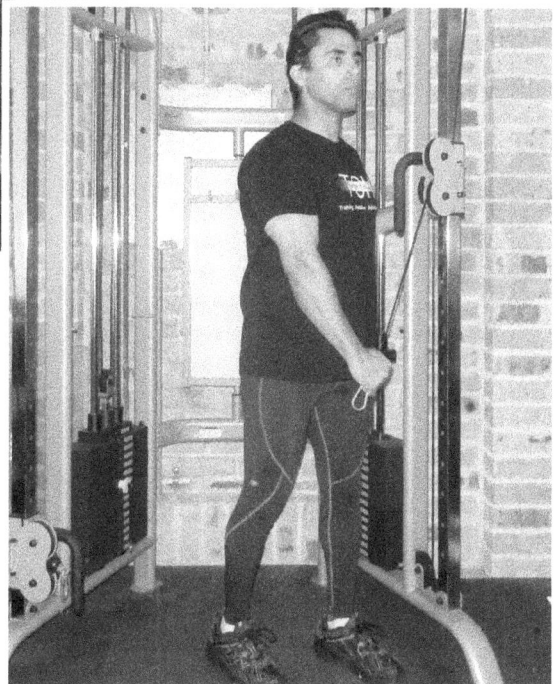

Finish:

Extend the working arm at the elbow joint, moving in a lateral direction to full extension.

(*Note:* Though it may not be evident in the photographs, the opposing hand must be secured to a stable structure.)

Standing: Long Head – Inferior Aspect

Start:

Adopt a unilateral stance (see page 47 for an explanation). Secure the opposing hand to a stable structure, with the working arm at 90° and slightly abducted. Grab the stirrup with the working hand in a semi-supine position.

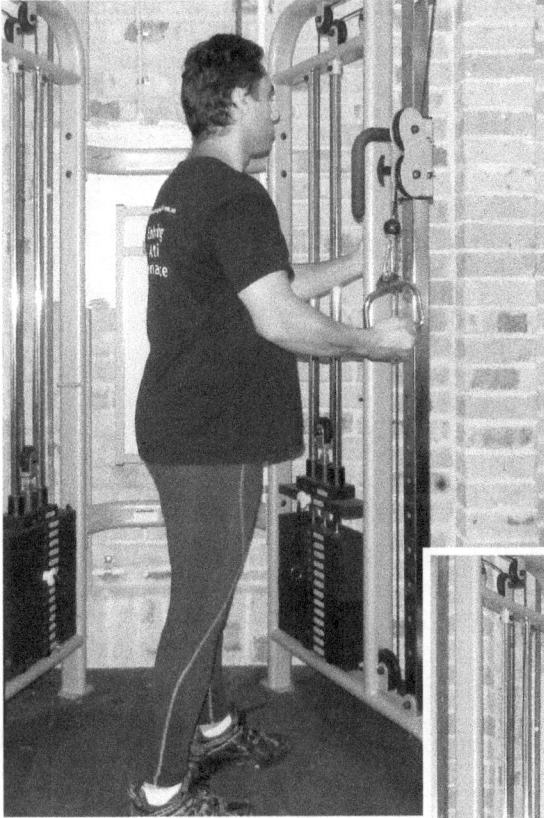

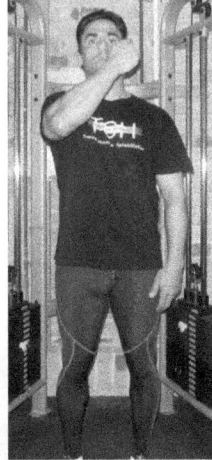

Front view

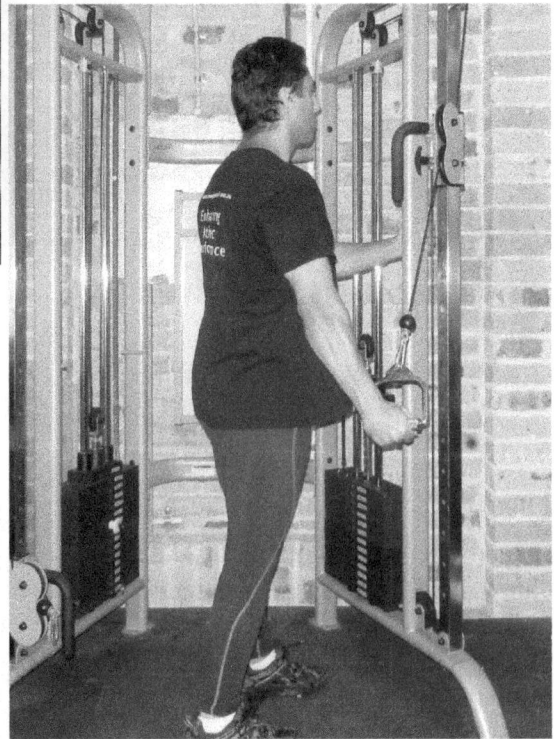

Finish:

Extend the working the arm at the elbow joint, moving in a lateral direction to full extension.

Standing: Medial Head

Start:

Adopt a unilateral stance (see page 47 for an explanation). Secure the opposing hand to a stable structure, with the working arm at 90° and adducted. Grab the stirrup with the working hand in a supine position.

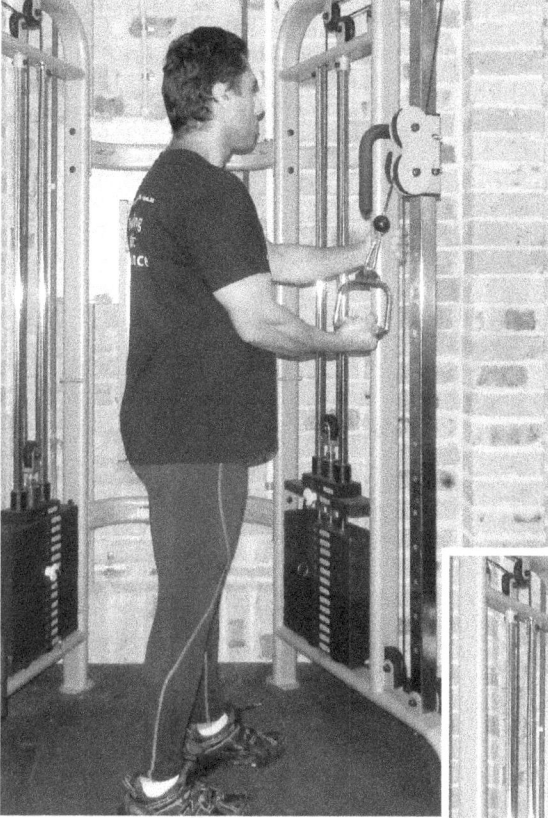

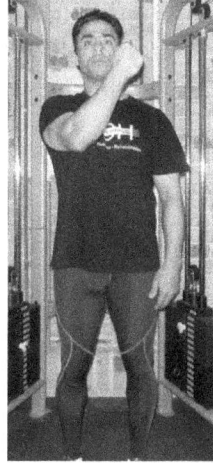

Front view

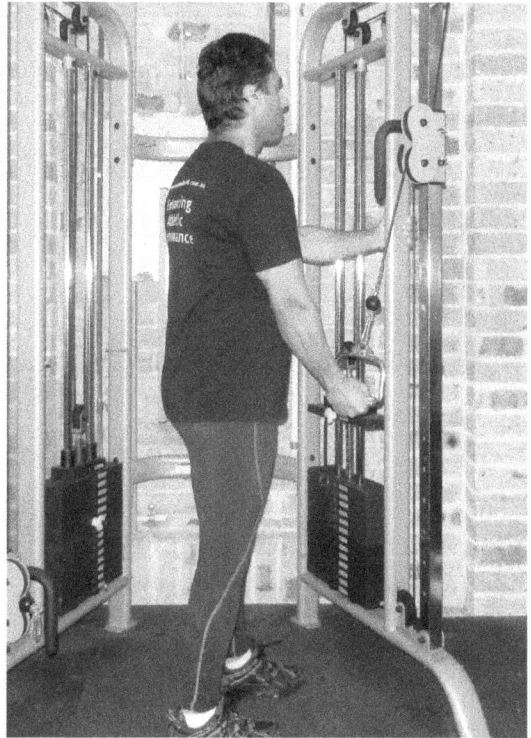

Finish:

Extend the working the arm at the elbow joint, moving in a lateral direction to full extension.

CABLE-PULLEY ADDUCTOR

Standing: Long Head – Superior Aspect

Start:

Adopt a unilateral stance (see page 47 for an explanation). Secure the opposing hand to a stable structure, then slightly abduct the working arm at the shoulder joint and bend at the elbow joint, so that the forearm and biceps contact. Grab the stirrup with the working hand in a semi-supine position.

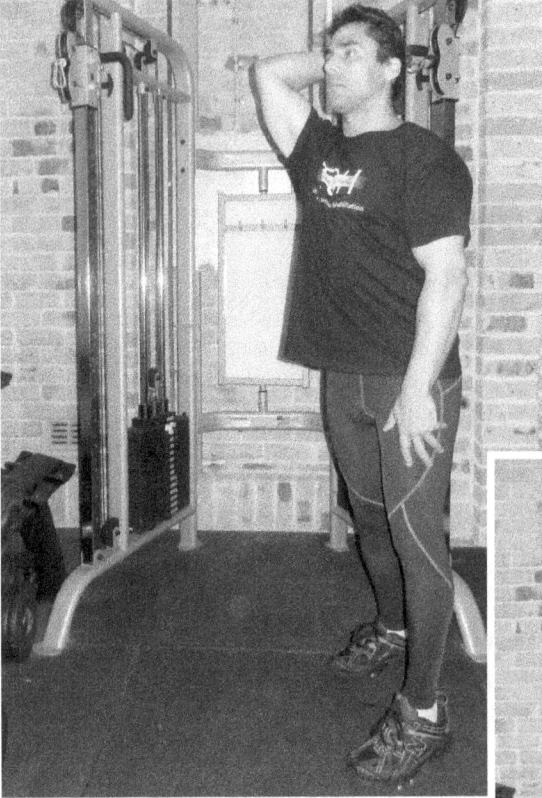

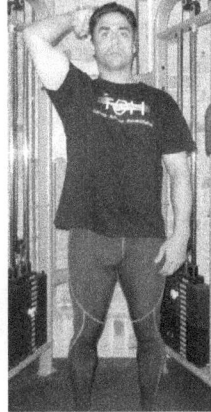

Front view

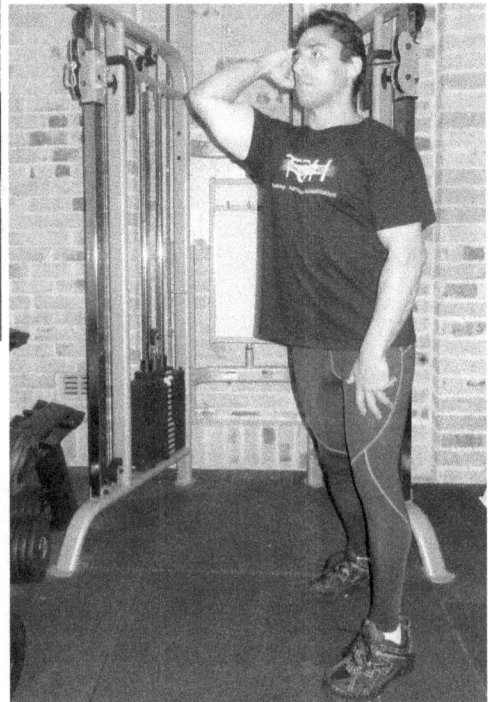

Finish:

Adduct the working arm at the shoulder joint, moving in a medial direction to the point where the elbow is pointing straight ahead.

(*Note:* Though not evident in the photographs, the opposing hand must be secured to a stable structure.)

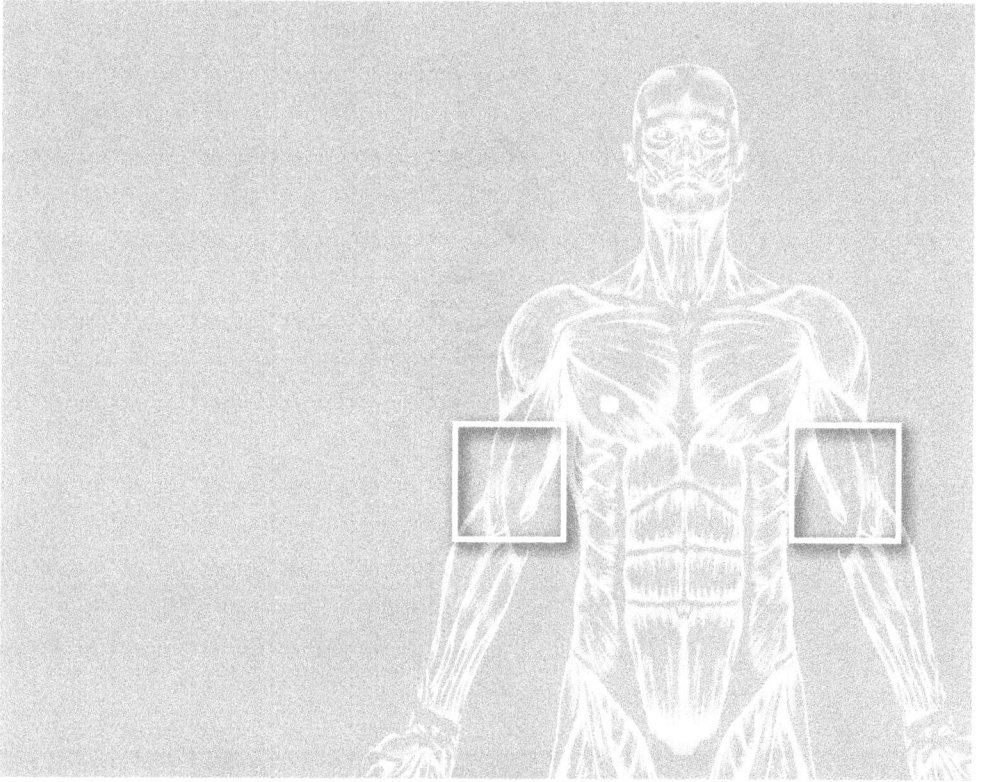

Brachialis Muscle Exercises

Brachialis

The brachialis are upper arm muscles positioned beneath the biceps muscles. They function to create flexion of the forearm at the elbow joint.

Figure 13.7 Brachialis muscle

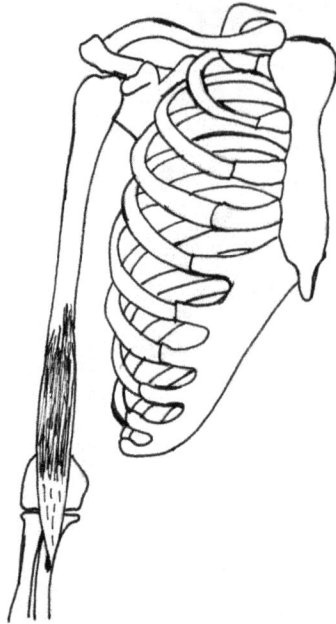

ORIGIN ATTACHMENT	INSERTION ATTACHMENT
• **Humerus** (front, lower half)	• **Ulna** (coronoid process, ulna tuberosity)

Things to consider:

☑ Isolation of the brachialis muscle is best achieved by placing the hand in a semi-prone position; this action rotates the radius bone to place it on top of the ulna bone. This relaxes the biceps muscle, minimising its contribution to elbow joint flexion.

☑ Hand position for brachialis muscle exercises will be created via the elbow and shoulder joints.

DUMBBELL REVERSE CURL

Standing: Whole Aspect

Start:

Adopt a unilateral stance (see page 47 for an explanation). Secure the opposing hand to a stable structure. Grab the dumbbell with the working hand in a semi-prone position.

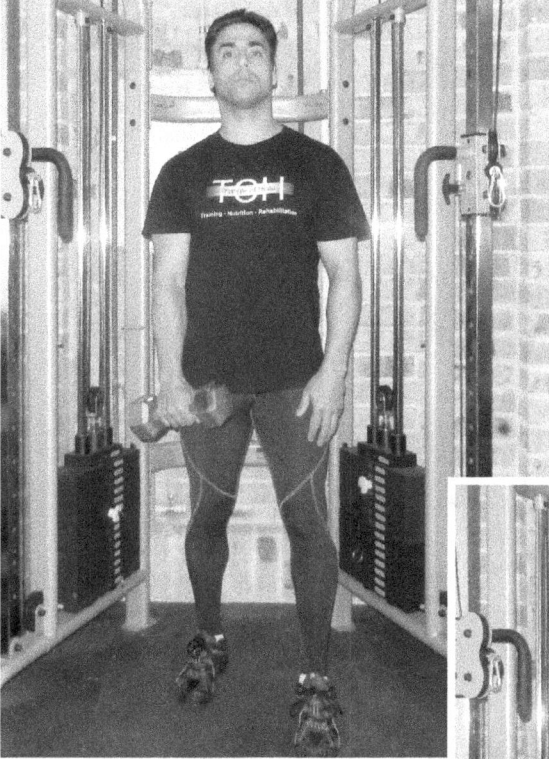

Finish:

Flex the working arm at the elbow joint, moving in a lateral direction reaching approximately 90°.

(*Note:* Though not evident in photographs, the opposing hand must be secured to a stable structure.)

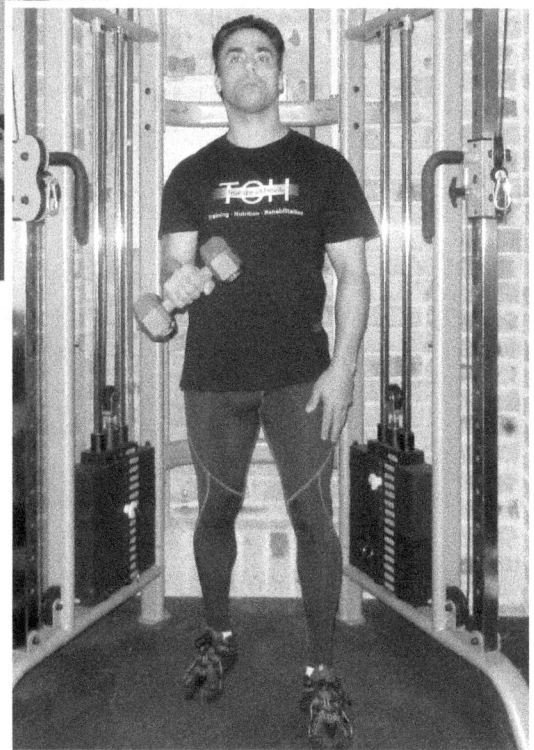

CABLE-PULLEY REVERSE CURL

Standing: Whole Aspect

Start:

Adopt a unilateral stance (see page 47 for an explanation). Secure the opposing hand to a stable structure. Grab the stirrup handle with the working hand in a semi-prone position.

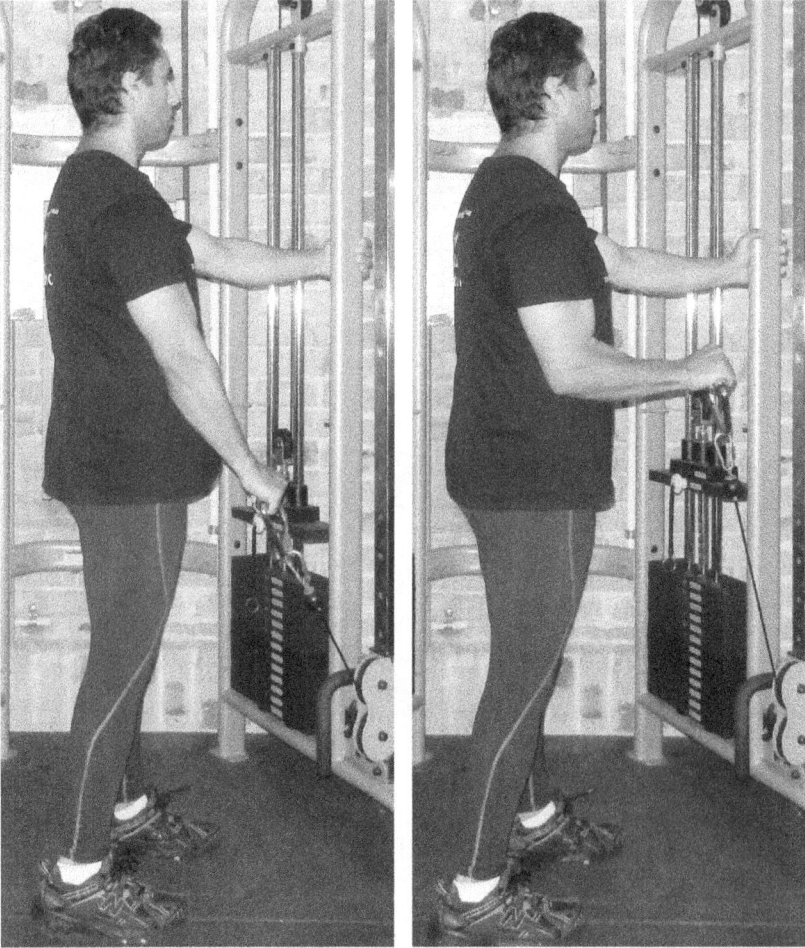

Finish:

Flex the working arm at the elbow joint, moving in a lateral direction reaching approximately 90°.

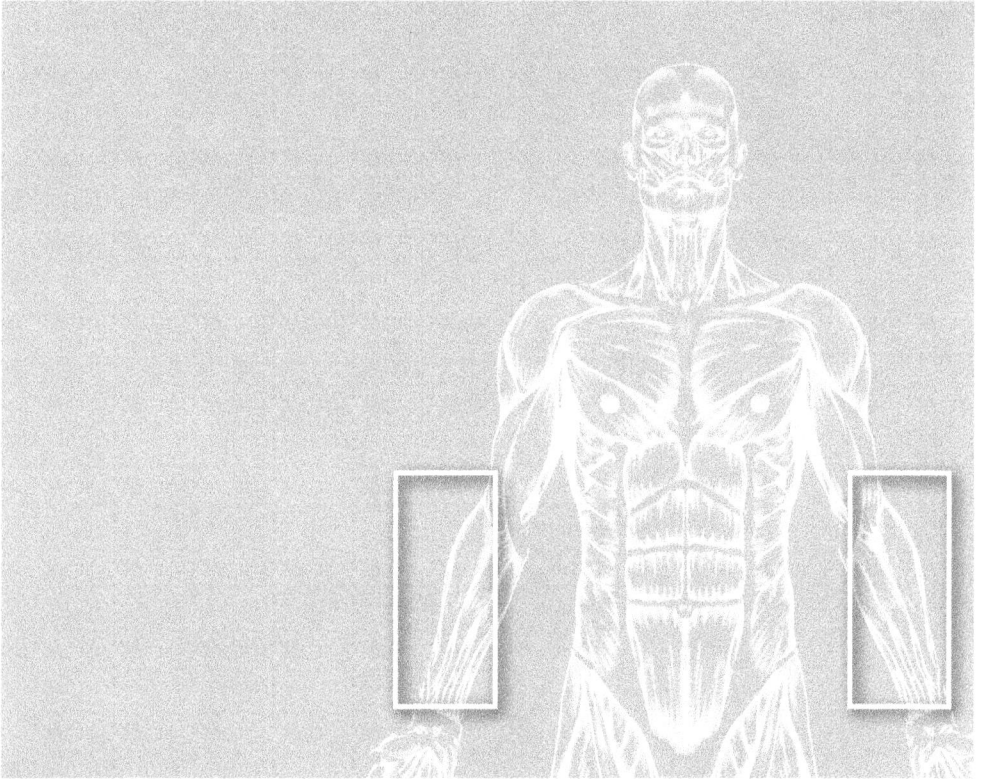

Brachioradialis Muscle Exercises

Brachioradialis

Positioned in the lower half of the arm, the brachioradialis muscles function to create flexion of the forearm at the elbow joint.

Figure 13.8 Brachioradialis muscle

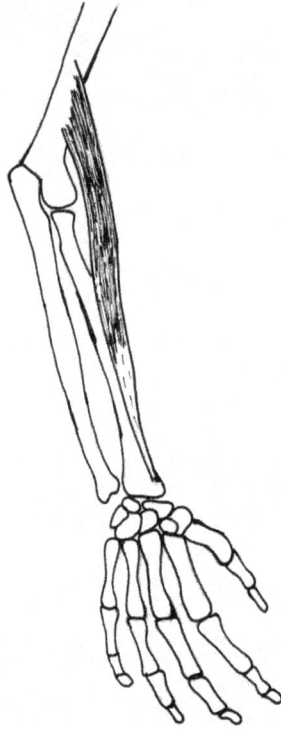

ORIGIN ATTACHMENT	INSERTION ATTACHMENT

• **Humerus**
  (lateral supracondylar ridge)
	• **Radius**
	  (styloid process base)

Things to consider:

☑ The brachioradialis is the strongest of the elbow joint flexor muscles.

☑ Exercises are executed with the hand in a neutral position, thumb pointing upward.

☑ Aesthetically, the brachioradialis accentuates the appearance of the arm as a whole.

☑ Hand position for the brachioradialis muscle exercises is created via the elbow and shoulder joints.

DUMBBELL HAMMER CURL

Standing: Whole Aspect

Start:

Adopt a unilateral stance (see page 47 for an explanation). Secure the opposing hand to a stable structure. Grab the dumbbell with the working hand in a neutral (thumb-up) position.

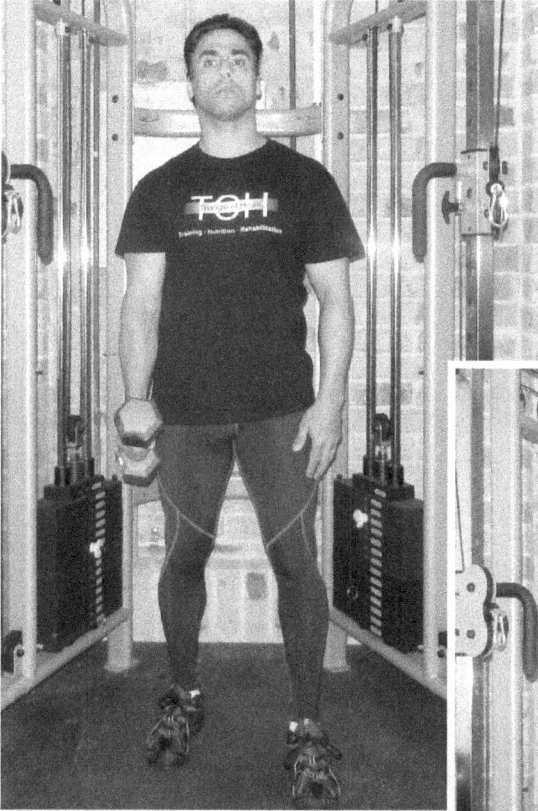

Finish:

Flex the working arm at the elbow joint, moving in a lateral direction reaching approximately 90°.

(*Note:* Though not evident in photographs, the opposing hand must be secured to a stable structure.)

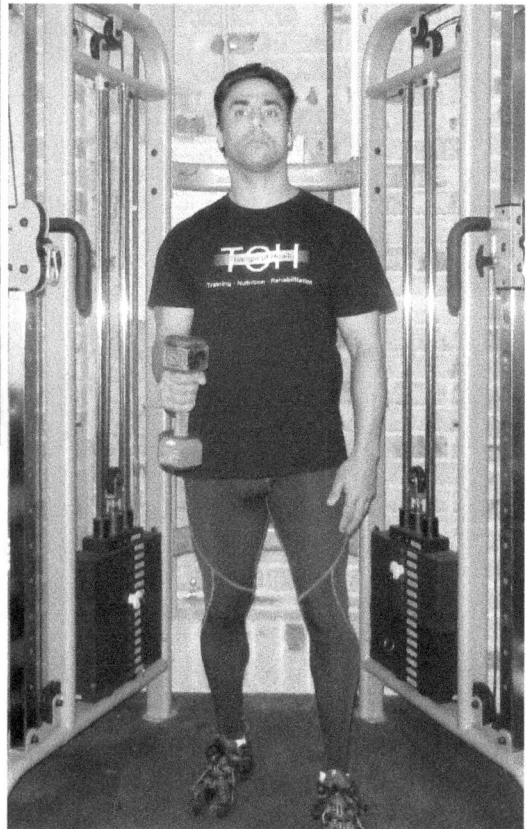

CABLE-PULLEY HAMMER CURL

Standing: Whole Aspect

Start:

Adopt a unilateral stance (see page 47 for an explanation). Secure the opposing hand to a stable structure. Grab the end of the cable with the working hand in a neutral (thumb-up) position.

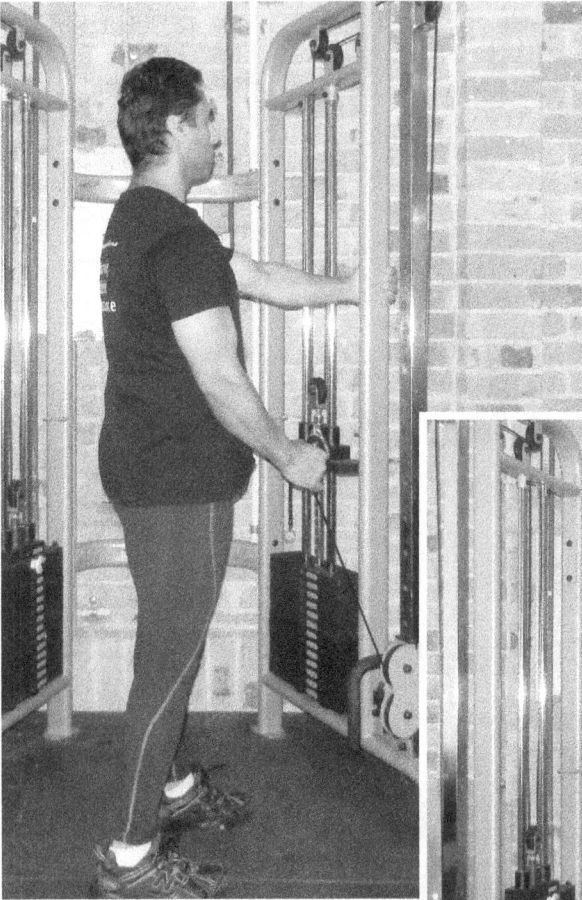

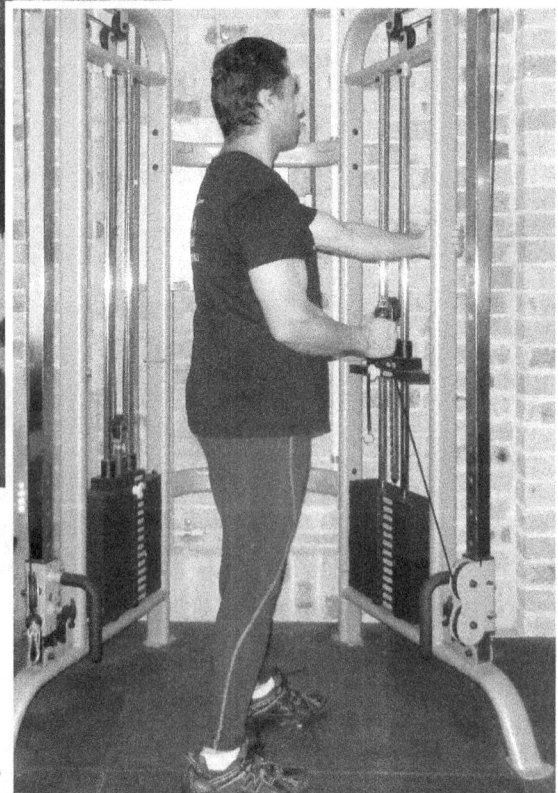

Finish:

Flex the working arm at the elbow joint, moving in a lateral direction reaching approximately 90°.

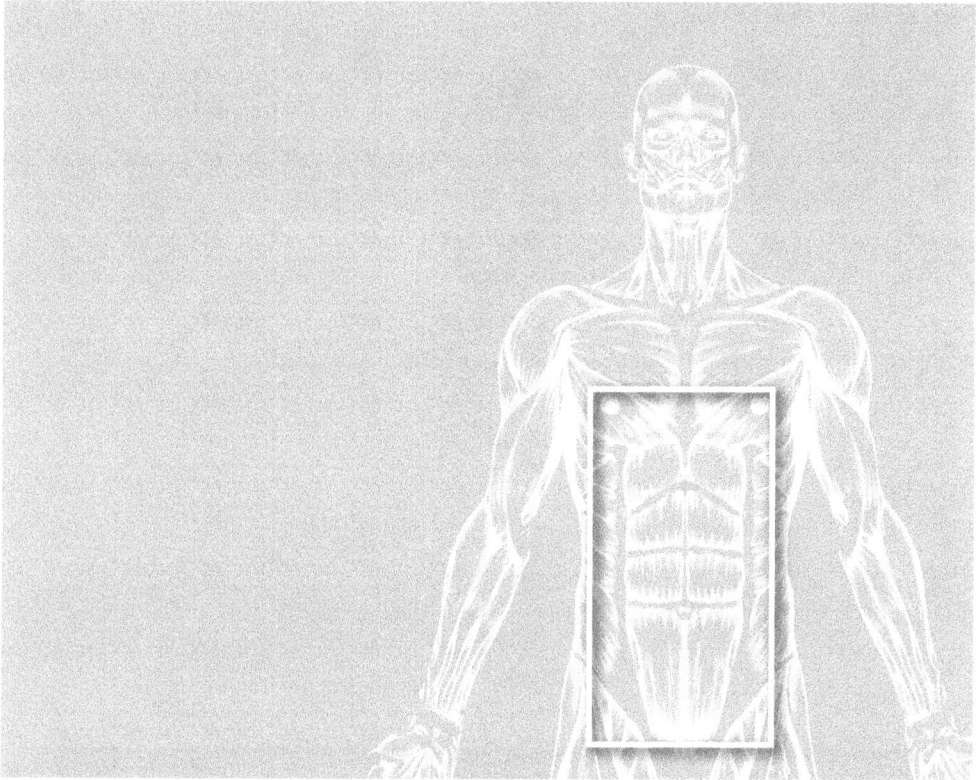

Rectus Abdominis Muscle Exercises

Rectus Abdominis

The rectus abdominis – or abdominal muscle commonly known as the 'abs' due to its composition of multiple heads – is a trunk muscle. It is separated left and right (mid-line of the body) by the linea alba, connective tissue composed of collagen, which runs down the middle of the abdomen.

The rectus abdominis muscle functions to create bending of the spine and compression of the abdominal area.

Figure 13.9 Rectus abdominis muscle

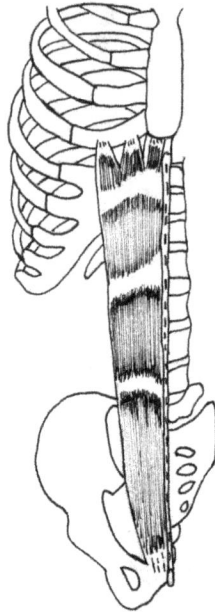

ORIGIN ATTACHMENT	INSERTION ATTACHMENT
• **Pelvis** (crest of pubic bone, pubic symphysis)	• **Cartilage** (ribs 5 – 7) • **Sternum** (xiphoid process)

Things to consider:

☑ A strong abdominal muscle helps to maintain the structural integrity of the back.

☑ To create greater isolation of the abdominal muscle, maintain the legs in an adducted position so that the hip flexor muscles (psoas, iliacus) are not used during the exercise.

☑ Lower muscle fibres are best isolated for exercise by placing the legs in an extended position, while upper fibres are best isolated in a bent-leg position.

☑ Contraction of the abdominal muscle is best executed in a rolling or curling type action: tucking the chin in and maintaining arms inward.

☑ Sit-up exercises cater to the opposite movements of back extension exercises.

SIT-UP

Supine: Straight Legs – Inferior Aspect

Start:

Lie supine with the legs straight, adducted and secured under a structurally sound piece of equipment, with arms extended and placed on top of the legs.

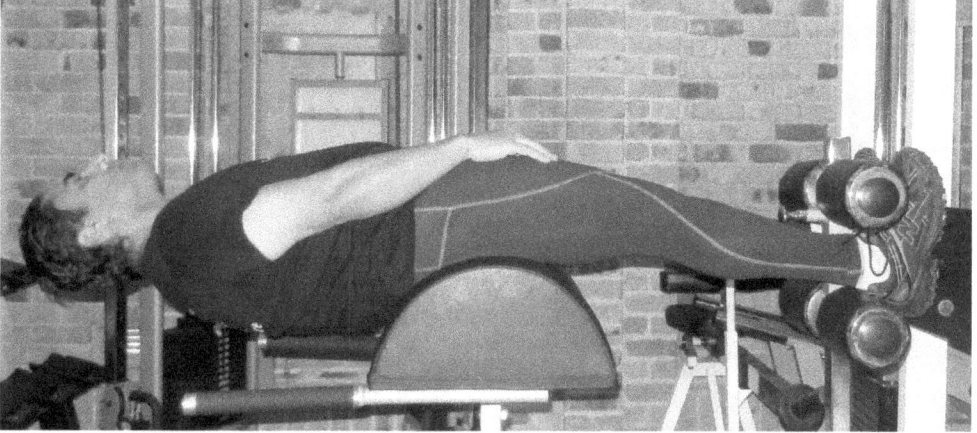

Finish:

With chin tucked in, flex the upper body in a forward direction short of 90°.

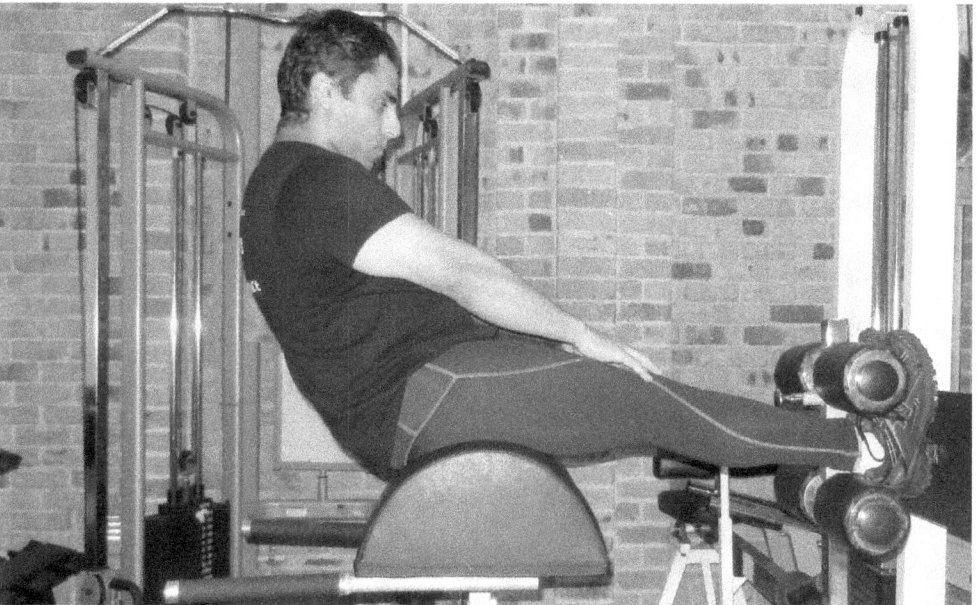

(*Note:* The machine is used for demonstration purposes. Exercise can be executed on the floor, as long as feet are secured.)

Supine: Bent Legs – Superior Aspect

Start:

Lie supine with the legs adducted, bent at the knee and hip joints and secured under a structurally sound piece of equipment, with arms extended and placed on top of the legs.

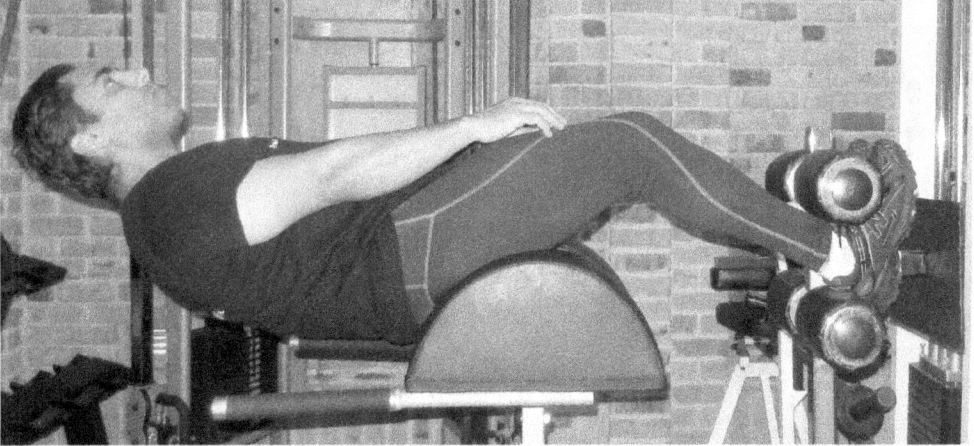

Finish:

With chin tucked in, flex the upper body in a forward direction short of 90°.

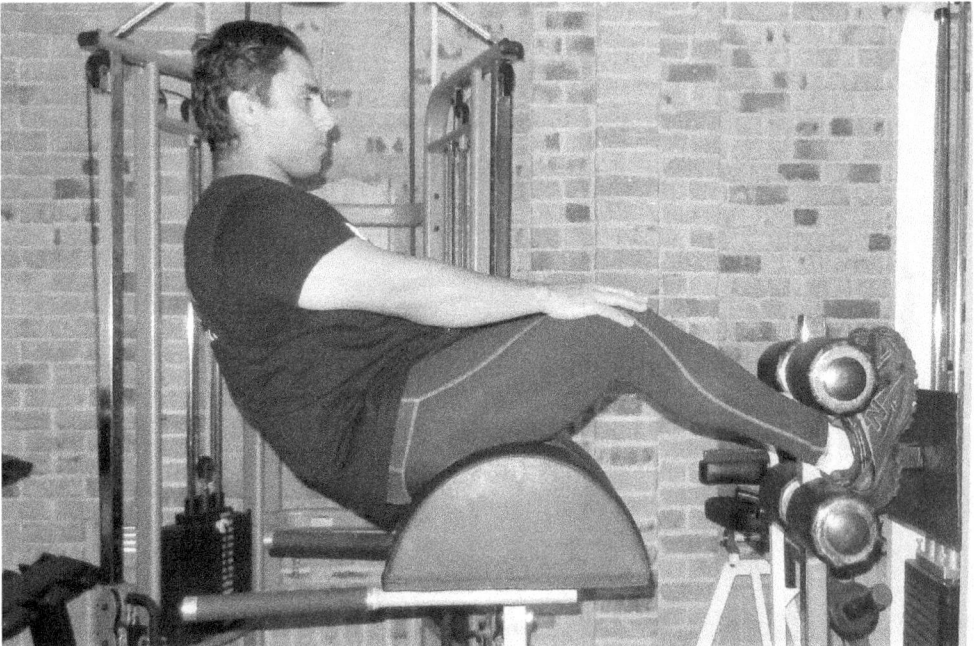

(*Note:* The machine is used for demonstration purposes. Exercise can be executed on the floor, as long as feet are secured.)

CRUNCH

Supine: Straight Legs – Inferior Aspect

Start:

Lie supine with the legs straight and adducted, with arms extended and placed on top of the legs.

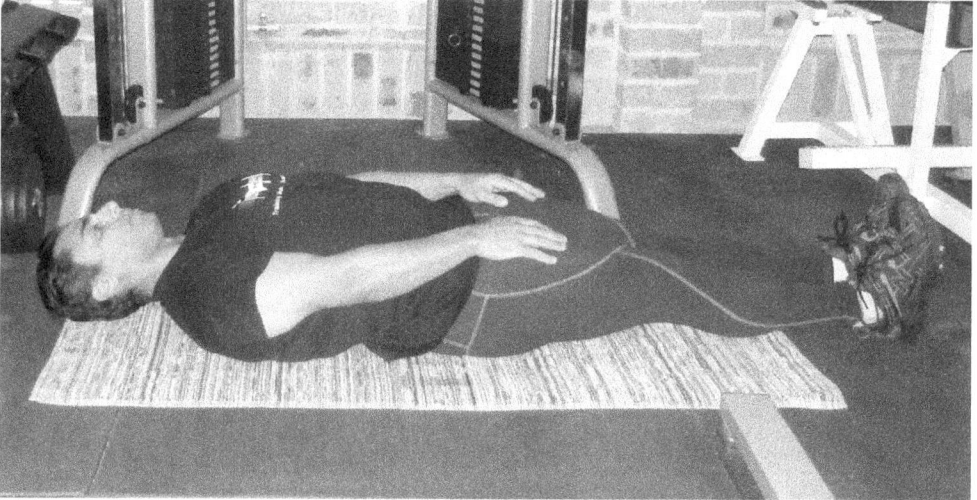

Finish:

With chin tucked in, flex the upper body in a slight forward direction.

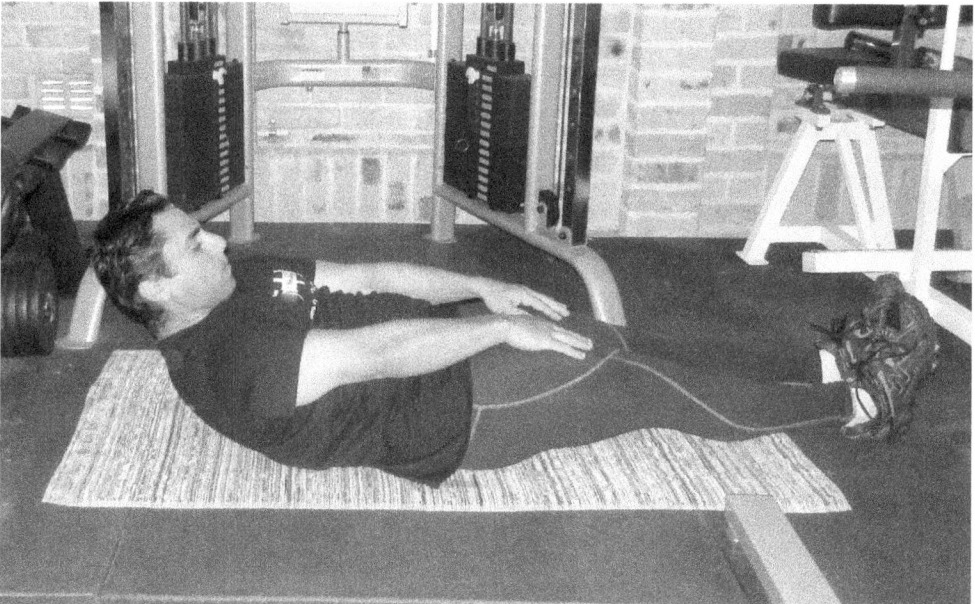

Supine: Bent Legs – Superior Aspect

Start:

Lie supine with the legs adducted and bent at the knee and hip joints, with arms extended placed on top of the legs.

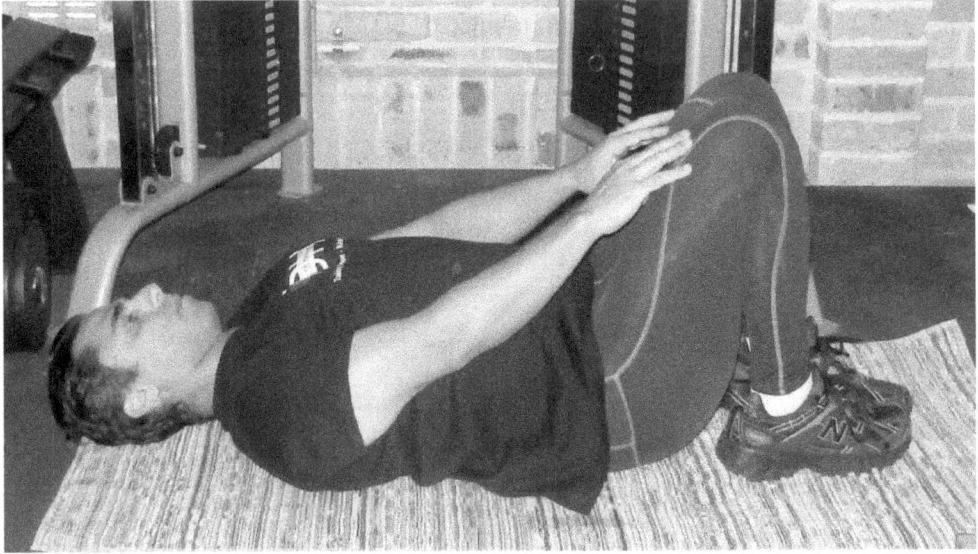

Finish:

With chin tucked in, flex the upper body in a slight forward direction.

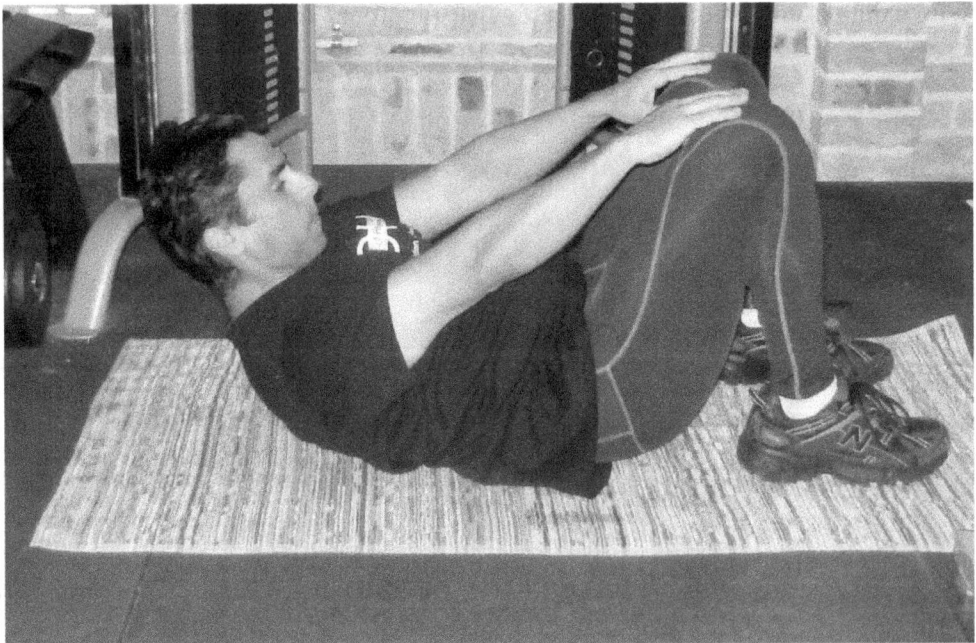

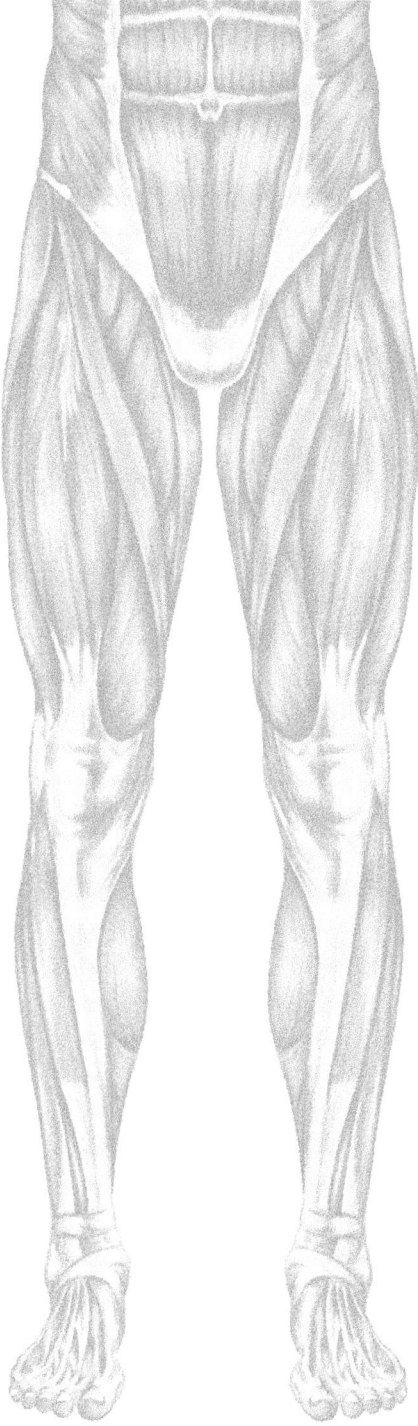

LOWER BODY

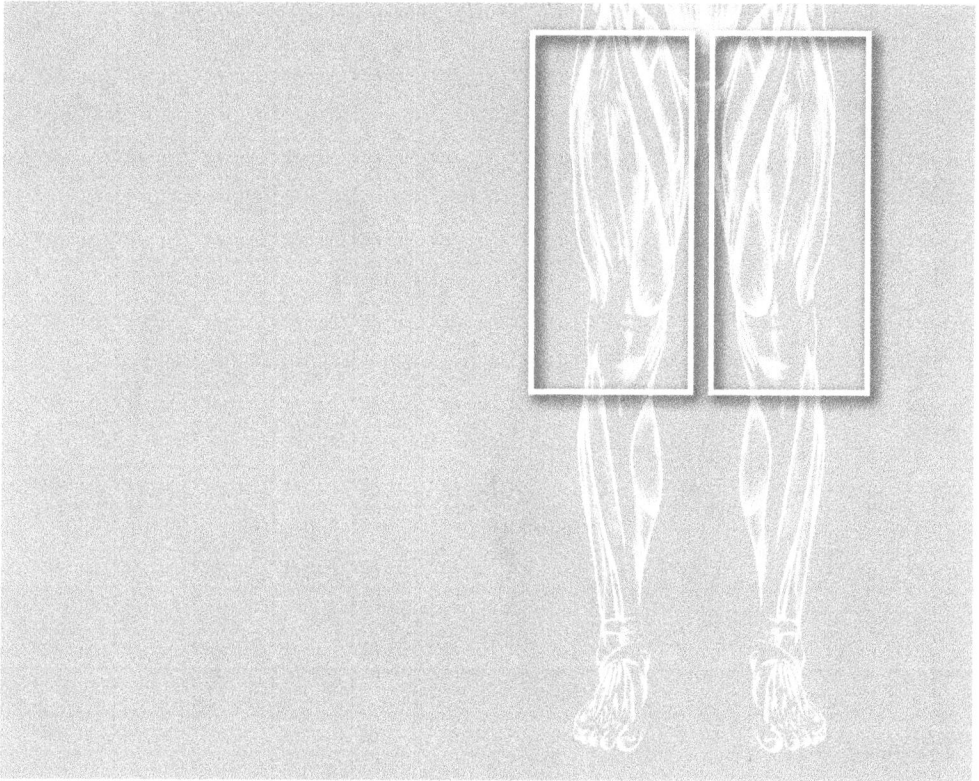

Quadricep Muscle Exercises

Quadriceps

The quadriceps, commonly known as the quads, are the biggest and strongest of the thigh muscles and occupy the front of the thigh. Each quadricep muscle is made up of four different heads:

- *vastus lateralis:* the most lateral and largest of the four heads

- *vastus medialis:* the most medial of the four heads

- *vastus intermedius:* the deepest of the four heads, situated underneath the rectus femoris

- *rectus femoris:* made up of the anterior (medial) and posterior (lateral) heads, and positioned between the vastus lateralis and medialis, above the intermedius.

All four heads of the quadricep muscle function to extend the lower leg at the knee joint, with the exception of the rectus femoris which also flexes the leg at the hip joint.

Figure 13.10 Quadricep muscle (a) vastus lateralis   (b) vastus intermedius   (c) vastus medialis
(d) rectus femoris (anterior)   (e) rectus femoris (posterior)

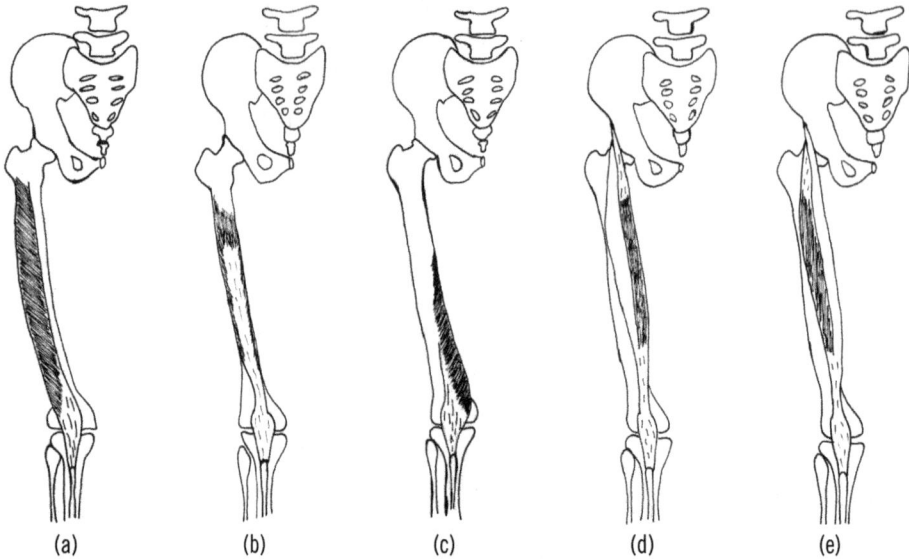

(a)   (b)   (c)   (d)   (e)

ORIGIN ATTACHMENT	INSERTION ATTACHMENT
Vastus lateralis • **Femur** (intertrochanteric line, greater trochanter, gluteal tuberosity)	• **Tibia** (tibial tuberosity)
Vastus intermedius • **Femur** (front, outer surface of upper two-thirds; linea aspera, lateral section of supracondylar line) • **Intrermuscular septum** (outer section)	• **Tibia** (tibial tuberosity)
Vastus medialis • **Femur** (medial aspect of linea aspera, medial section of supracondylar line) • **Intermuscular septum** (inner section)	• **Tibia** (tibial tuberosity, medial condyle)
Rectus femoris (anterior) • **Pelvis** (anterior inferior iliac spine)	• **Tibia** (tibial tuberosity)
Rectus femoris (posterior) • **Pelvis** (top part of acetabulum)	• **Tibia** (tibial tuberosity)

Things to consider:

☑ The function of the quadricep is not only movement but also protection and support of the knee joint.

☑ A caution: constant hyper-extension – fully locking out at the knee joint – will, over time, wear away the articulating cartilage and increase the risk of knee joint damage.

☑ Foot position for quadricep muscle exercises will be created via the hip and ankle joints and will vary depending on what aspect is exercised.

☑ Vastus medialis oblique, the bottom portion of the vastus medialis muscle (attached to the medial aspect of the kneecap), functions to carry out the last part of the extension of the lower leg by rotating the tibia on the femur.

☑ Flexing or raising of the leg at the hip joint will assist in greater activation of the vasti muscles (medialis, intermedius, lateralis) due to the shortening or slackening of the rectus femoris muscle, and vice versa.

MACHINE LEG EXTENSION

Seated: Vastus Medialis – Superior Aspect

Start:

Seated in a 90° position, abduct and laterally rotate the working leg at the hip joint, then evert and plantar flex the working foot. Secure the opposing foot, out of the way.

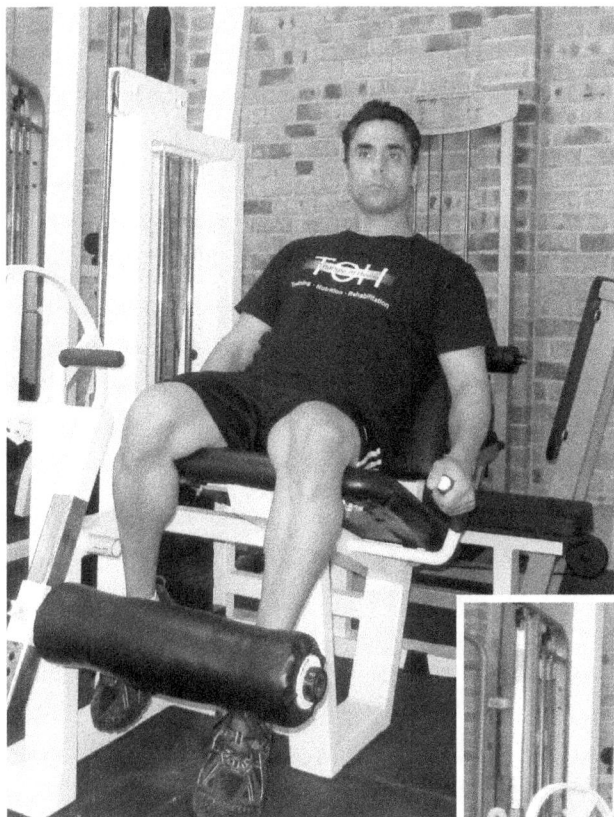

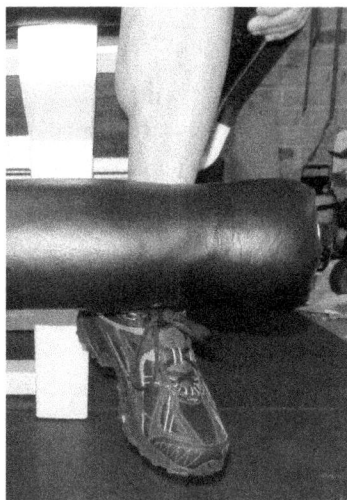

Everted and plantar flexed
(toes pointing outward and down)

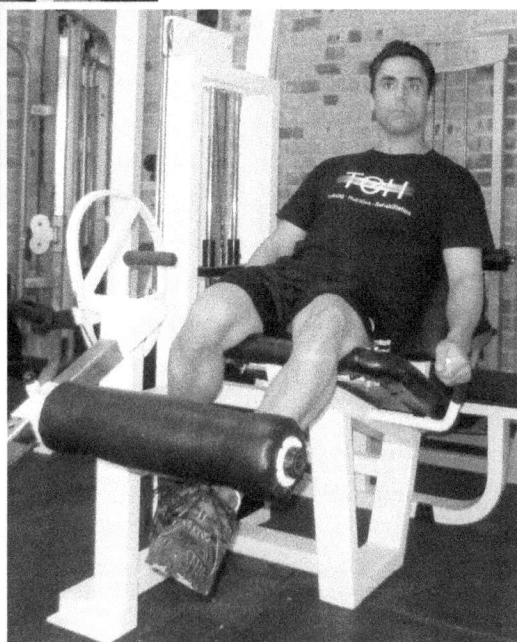

Finish:

Extend the lower half of the working leg at the knee joint, moving the foot in a medial direction short of hyper-extension.

Seated: Vastus Intermedius – Superior Aspect

Start:

Seated in a 90° position, with the working leg aligned between the knee and the hip joint, place the working foot in a neutral and dorsiflexed position. Secure the opposing foot, out of the way.

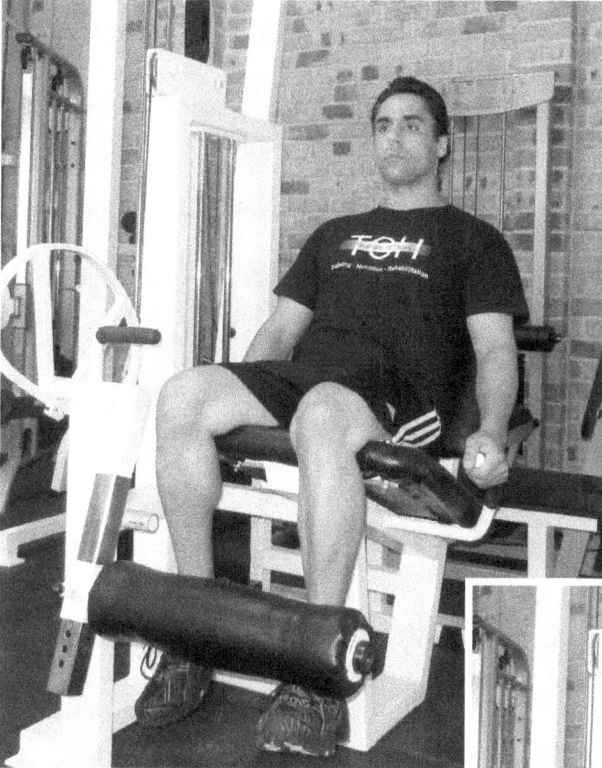

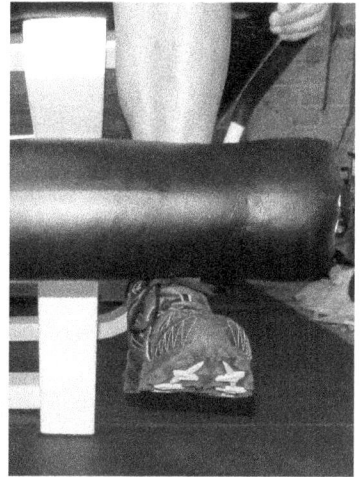

Neutral and dorsiflexed
(toes pointing forward and up)

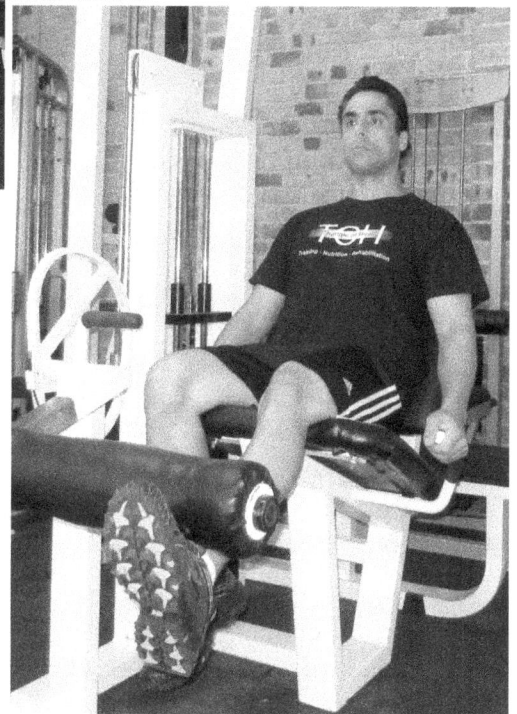

Finish:

Extend the lower half of the working leg at the knee joint, moving the foot in a forward direction short of hyper-extension.

Seated: Vastus Lateralis – Superior Aspect

Start:

Seated in a 90° position, adduct and medially rotate the working leg at the hip joint, then invert and dorsiflex the working foot. Secure the opposing foot, out of the way.

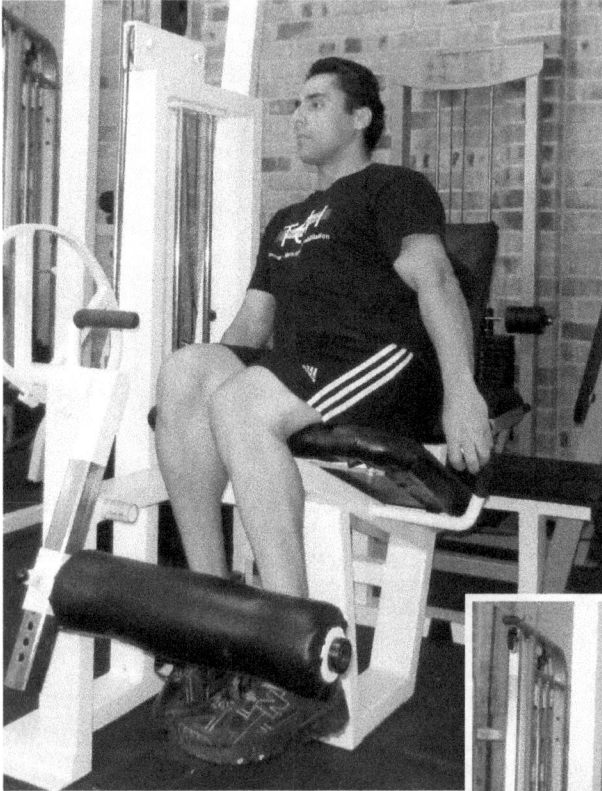

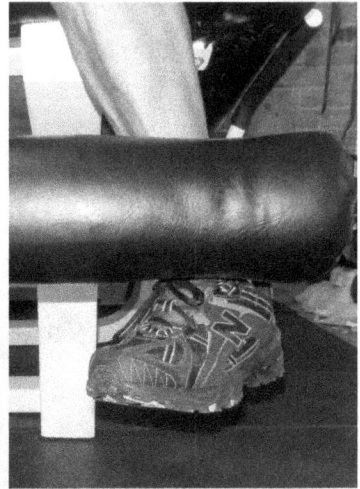

Inverted and dorsiflexed
(toes pointing inward and up)

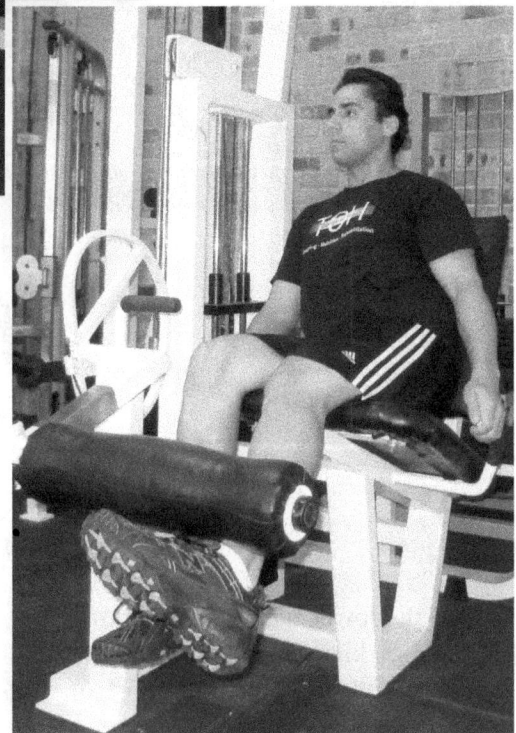

Finish:

Extend the lower half of the working leg at the knee joint, moving the foot in a lateral direction short of hyper-extension.

Standing: Vastus Medialis Oblique – Inferior Aspect

Start:

Standing upright with a hand secured to a stable structure, abduct and laterally rotate the leg at the hip joint, then evert and dorsiflex the working foot. Secure the opposing foot, out of the way.

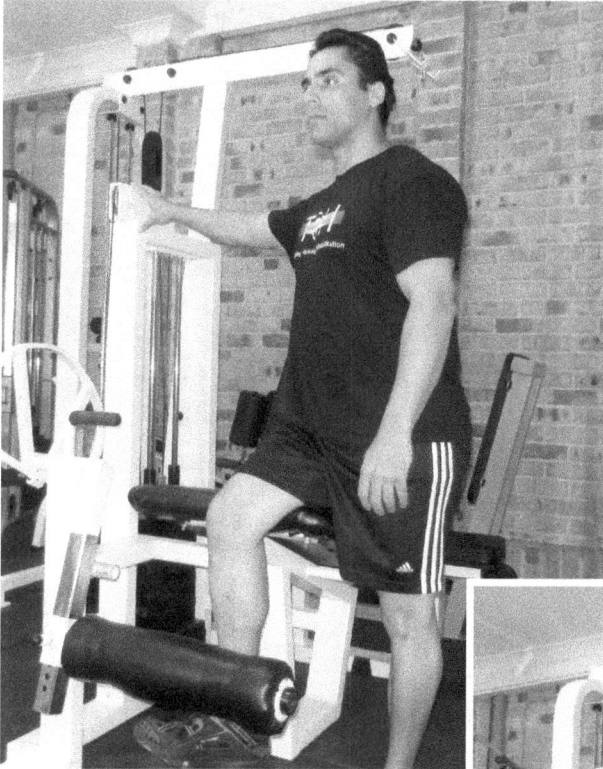

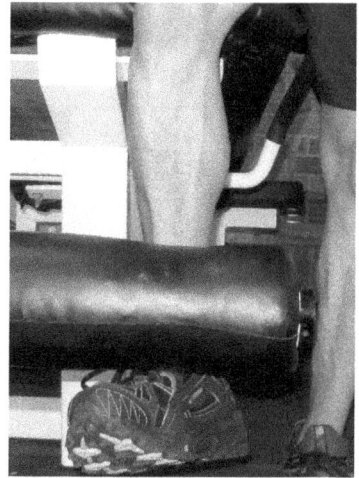

Everted and dorsiflexed
(toes pointing outward and up)

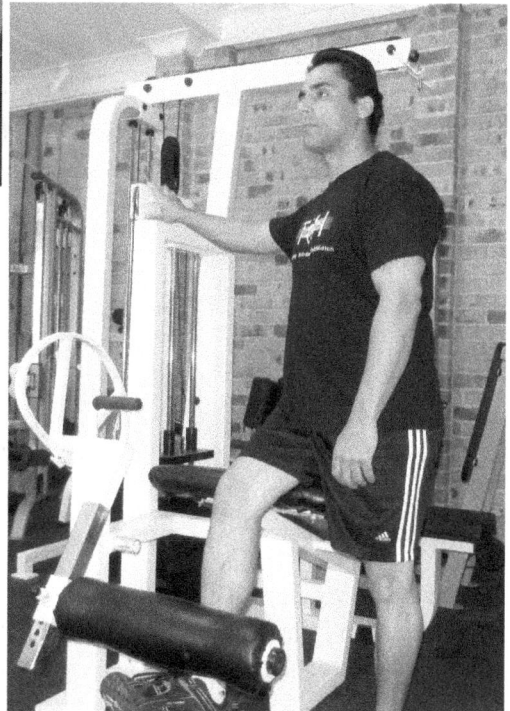

Finish:

Extend the lower half of the working leg at the knee joint, moving the foot in a medial direction short of hyper-extension.

Standing: Vastus Intermedius – Inferior Aspect

Start:

Standing upright, with a hand secured to a stable structure and with the working leg aligned between the knee and the hip joint, place the working foot in a neutral and plantar flexed position.

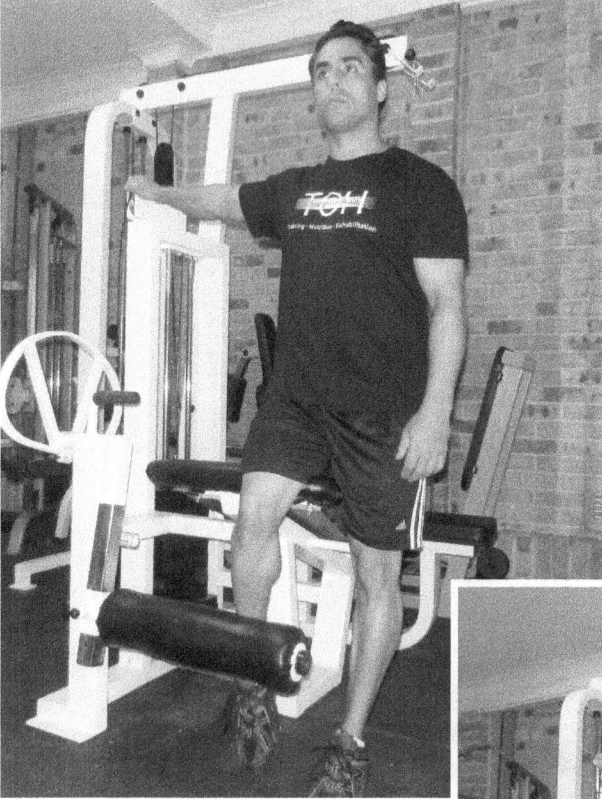

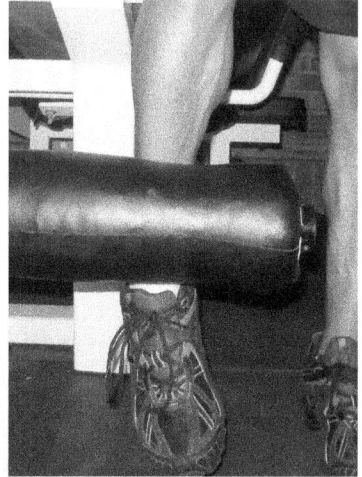

Neutral and plantar flexed
(toes pointing forward and down)

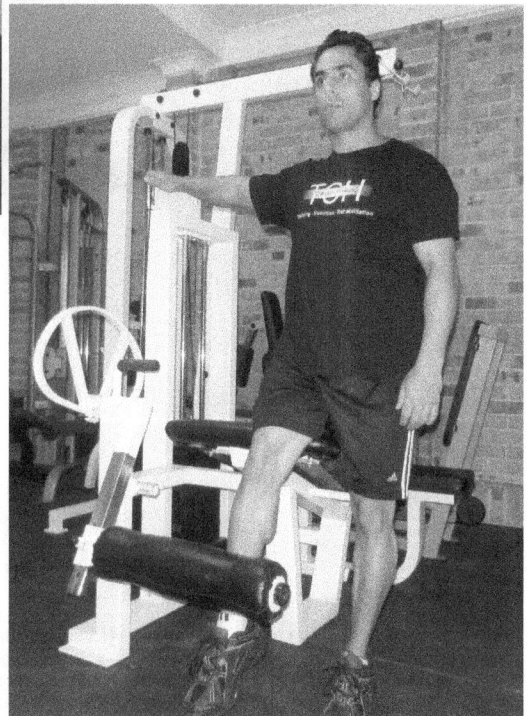

Finish:

Extend the lower half of the working leg at the knee joint, moving the foot in a forward direction short of hyper-extension.

Standing: Vastus Lateralis – Inferior Aspect

Start:

Standing upright, adduct and medially rotate the working leg at the hip joint, then invert and plantar flex the working foot.

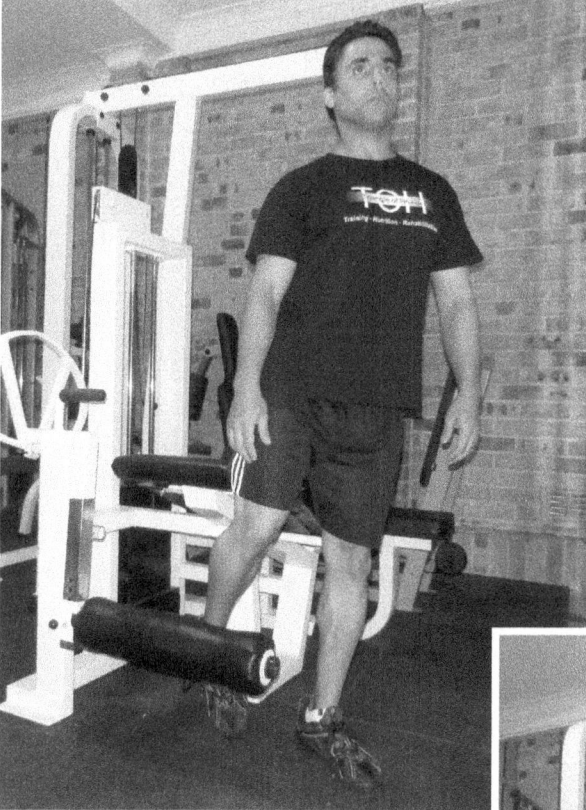

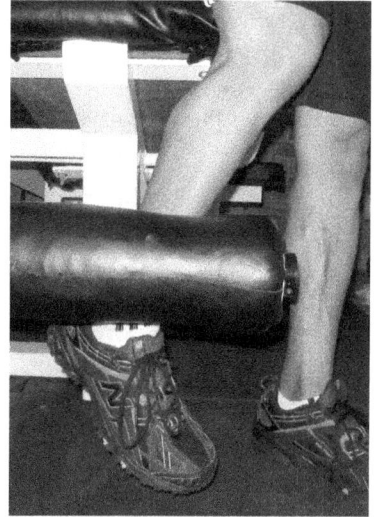

Inverted and plantar flexed
(toes pointing inward and down)

Finish:

Extend the lower half of the working leg at the knee joint, moving the foot in a lateral direction short of hyper-extension.

(*Note:* Though not evident in the photographs, secure the opposing hand to the closest machine or stable structure in the vicinity.)

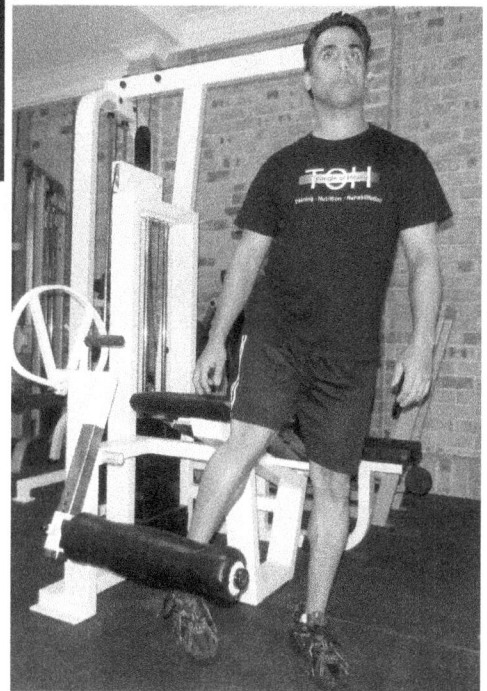

CABLE-PULLEY LEG FLEXION

Standing: Rectus Femoris – Anterior Head

Start:

Adopt a unilateral stance (see page 47 for an explanation) and secure the opposing hand onto a stable structure. Align the heel of the working leg with the toes of the opposing foot, and laterally rotate the leg at the hip joint so the working foot is everted, and then dorsiflex the foot.

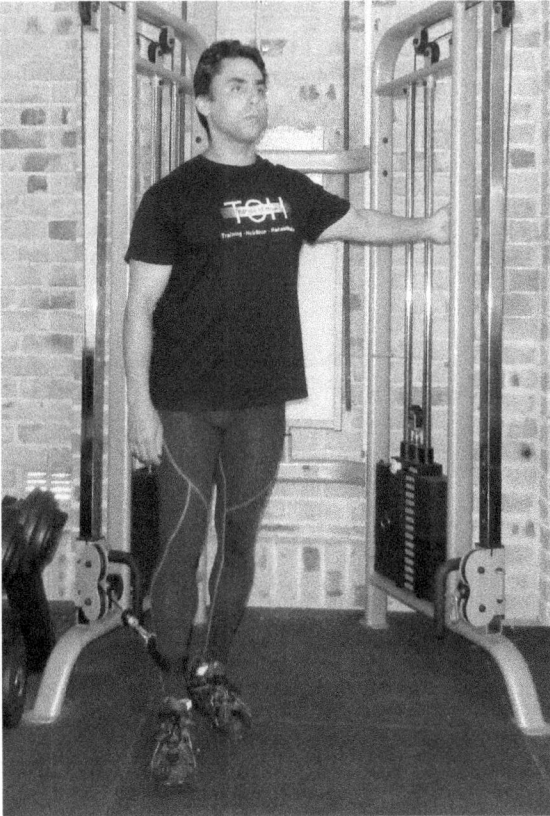

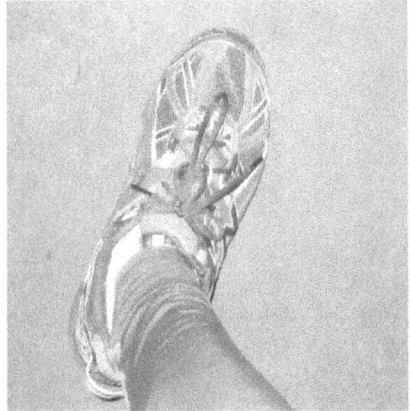

Everted
(toes pointing outward)

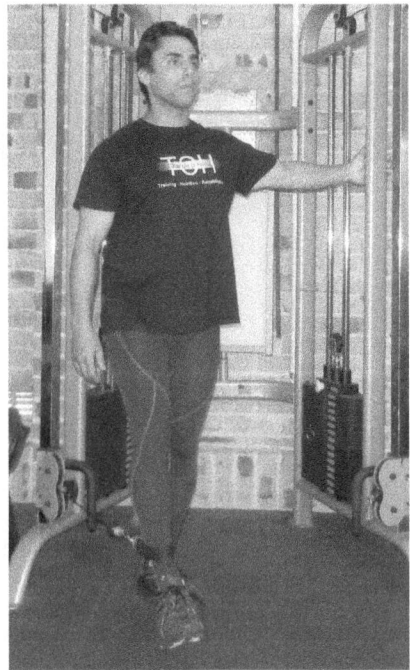

Finish:

Flex the working leg at the hip joint, moving the foot in a forward direction to the initial point of stoppage.

(*Note:* Some form of ankle strap will be required to execute this exercise.)

Standing: Rectus Femoris – Posterior Head

Start:

Adopt a unilateral stance (see page 47 for an explanation) and secure the opposing hand onto a stable structure. Align the heel of the working leg with the toes of the opposing foot, maintaining the working foot in a neutral and dorsiflexed position.

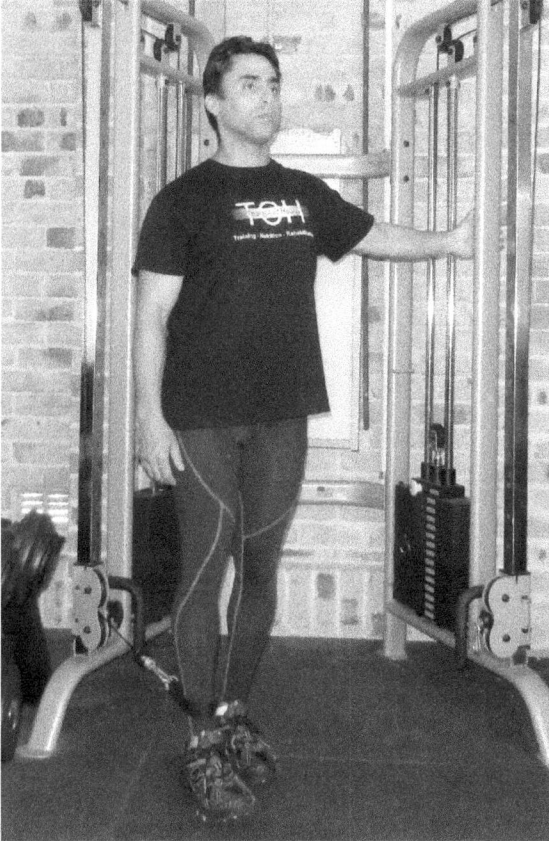

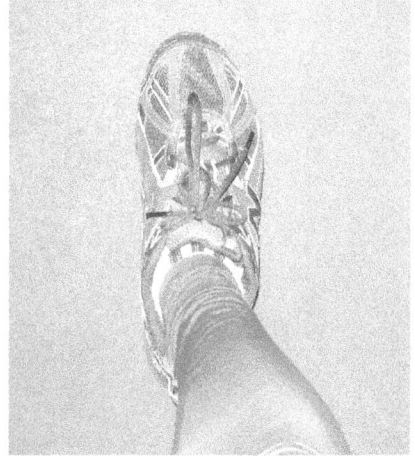

Neutral
(toes pointing forward)

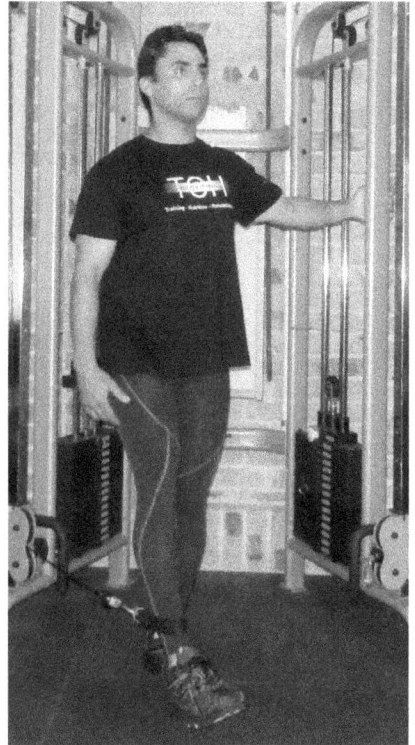

Finish:

Flex the working leg at the hip joint, moving the foot in a forward direction to the initial point of stoppage.

(*Note:* Some form of ankle strap will be required to execute this exercise.)

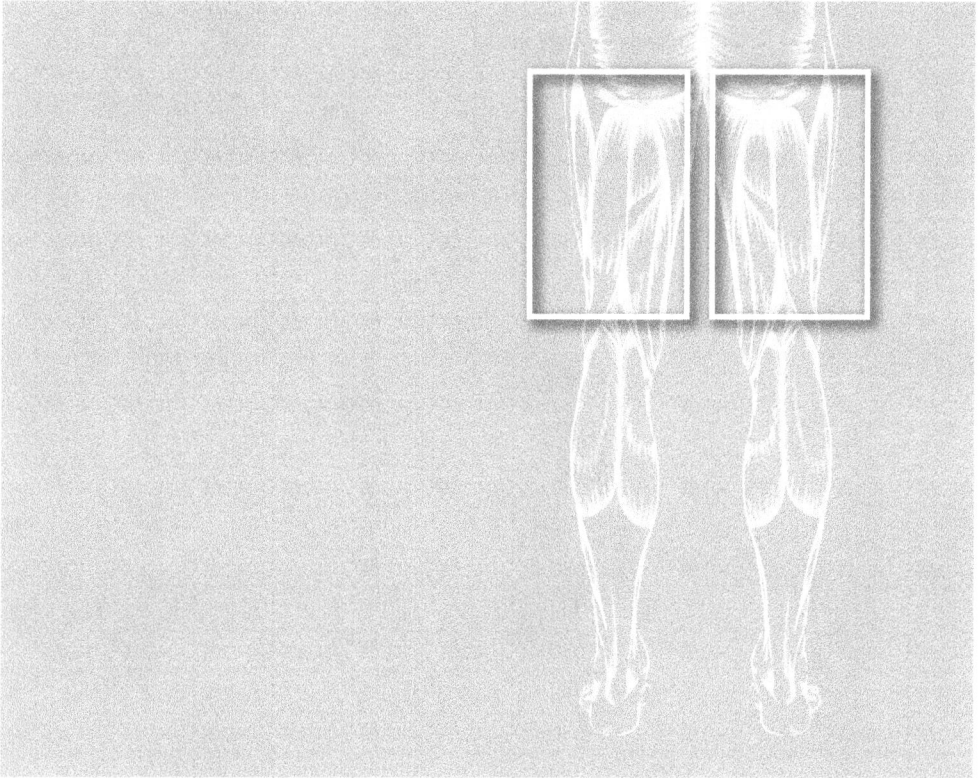

Hamstring Muscle Exercises

Hamstrings

The hamstring muscles are positioned to the rear of the quadriceps on the back of each thigh and are made up of three different muscles: biceps femoris, semitendinosus and semimembranosus. They function at the hip and knee joint to carry out three separate movements, as described below:

- *biceps femoris* – the largest and most lateral of the hamstring muscles, and made up of two heads. The short head functions only to flex the lower leg at the knee joint, and the long head is involved in knee joint flexion and extension of the leg at the hip joint.

- *semitendinosus* – part tendon, part muscle, it is situated medially and functions to create flexion and slight medial rotation of the lower leg at the knee joint and extension of the leg at the hip joint

- *semimembranosus* – part membrane, part muscle, it is situated medially and functions to create flexion and slight medial rotation of the lower leg at the knee joint and extension of the leg at the hip joint.

Figure 13.11 Hamstring muscle (a) biceps long head (b) biceps short head (c) semitendinosus
(d) semimembranosus

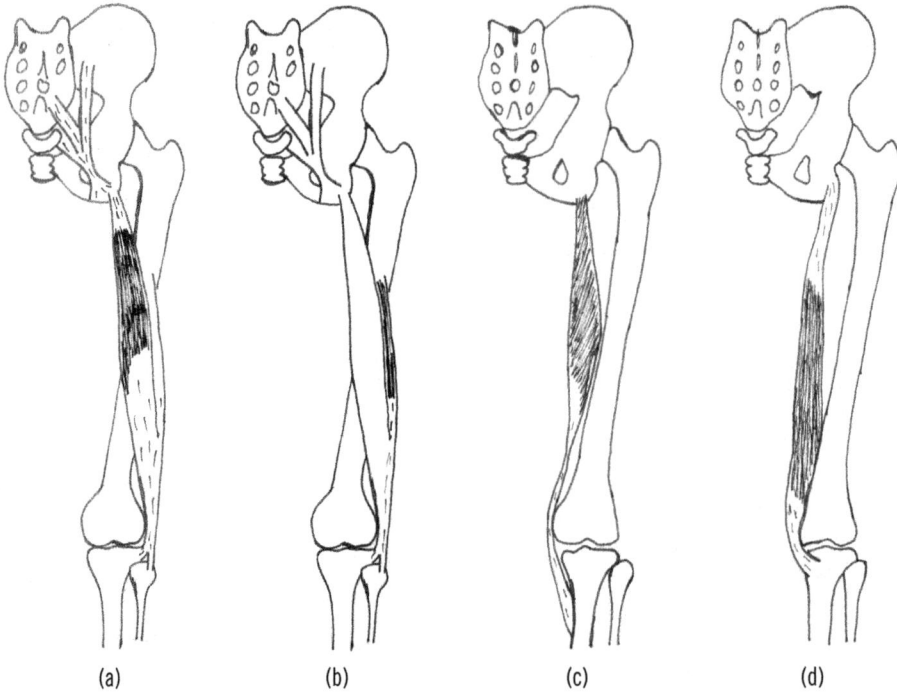

| (a) | (b) | (c) | (d) |

ORIGIN ATTACHMENT	INSERTION ATTACHMENT
Biceps femoris (long head) • **Pelvis** (ischial tuberosity, sacrotuberous ligament)	• **Tibia** (lateral aspect) • **Fibula** (lateral aspect)
Biceps femoris (short head) • **Femur** (linea aspera, lateral supracondylar ridge)	• **Tibia** (lateral aspect) • **Fibula** (lateral aspect)
Semitendinosus • **Pelvis** (ischial tuberosity)	• **Tibia** (medial shaft)
Semimembranosus • **Pelvis** (ischial tuberosity)	• **Tibia** (rear, medial condyle)

Things to consider:

☑ Foot position for hamstring muscle exercises will be created via the hip and ankle joints.

☑ Position of the hip, legs and feet will influence various sections and aspects of the hamstring muscles.

☑ Abducting, rotating the leg medially and inverting the foot isolates the medial aspect of the hamstring muscle in that leg; adducting, rotating the leg laterally and everting the foot isolates the lateral aspect of the hamstring.

☑ To avoid the gastrocnemius portion of the calf muscle contributing to knee joint flexion during hamstring exercises, dorsiflexion of the foot is necessary.

☑ Flexion of the leg at the hip joint allows greater isolation of the biceps femoris short head.

☑ Weakness of the hamstring muscles can contribute to issues related to pelvic instability and back pain.

MACHINE LEG CURL

Prone: Superior – Lateral Aspect

Start:

Lie prone, raise the pelvis, adduct and laterally rotate the working leg, evert and dorsiflex the foot, then flex the working leg at the knee joint at 90°.

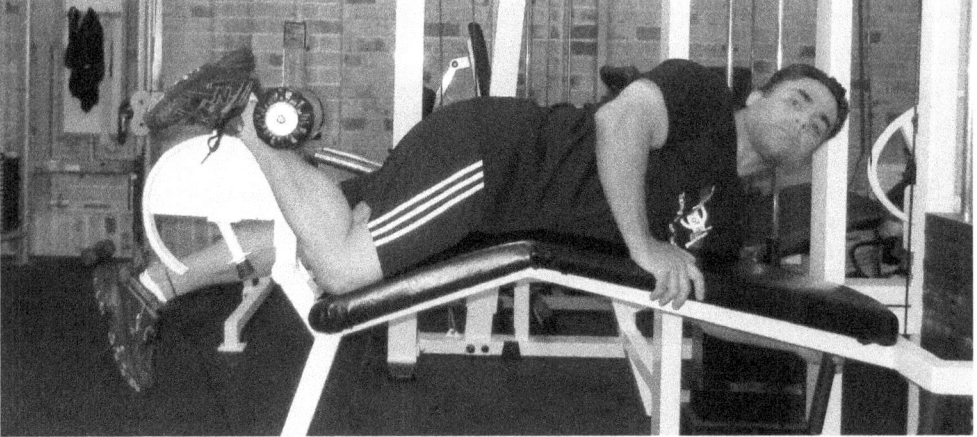

Finish:

Flex the lower half of the working leg at the knee joint, moving the foot in a lateral direction to initial contact of calf and hamstring muscle in that leg.

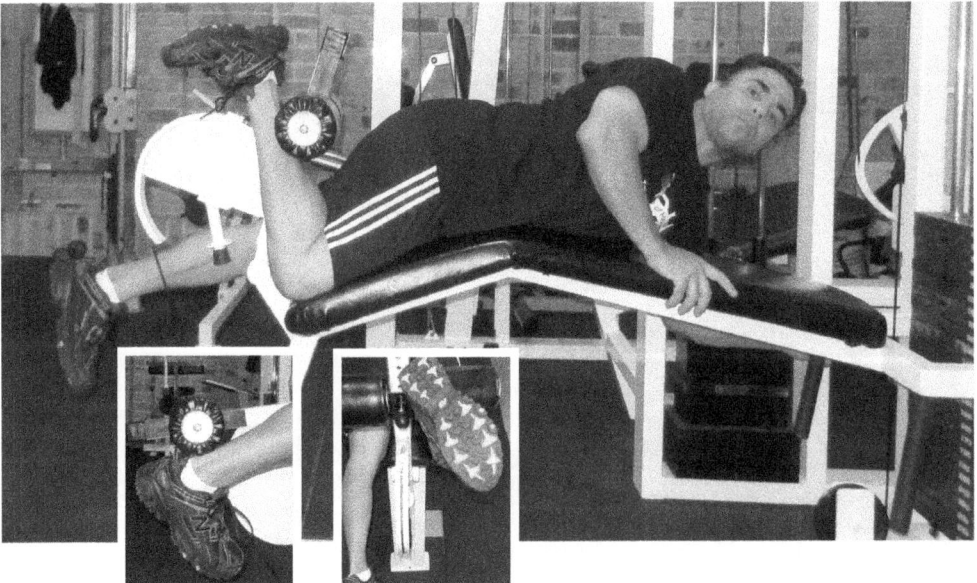

Dorsiflexed
(toes upward)

Everted
(toes outward)

Prone: Superior – Middle Aspect

Start:

Lie prone, pelvis against the machine, the working leg aligned with the knee and the hip joint, the foot neutral and dorsiflexed, then flex the working leg at the knee joint at 90°.

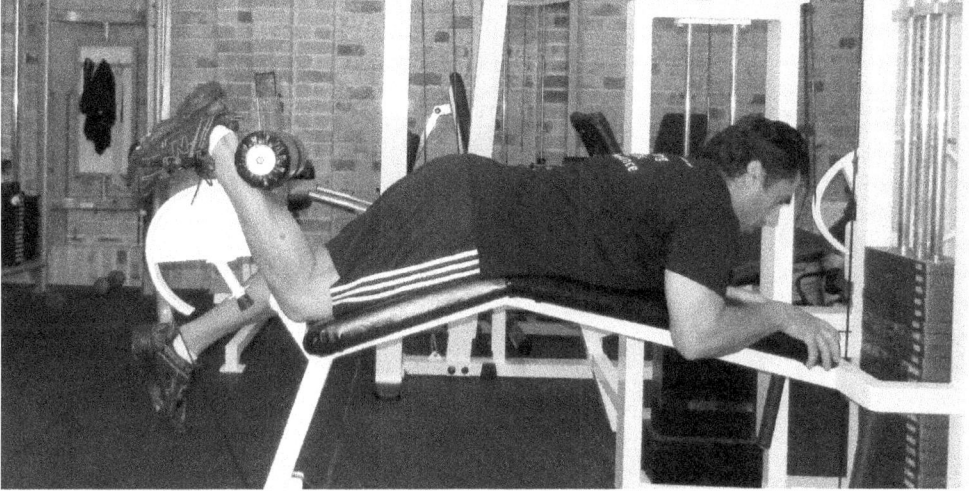

Finish:

Flex the lower half of the working leg at the knee joint, moving the foot in a forward direction to initial contact of calf and hamstring muscle in that leg.

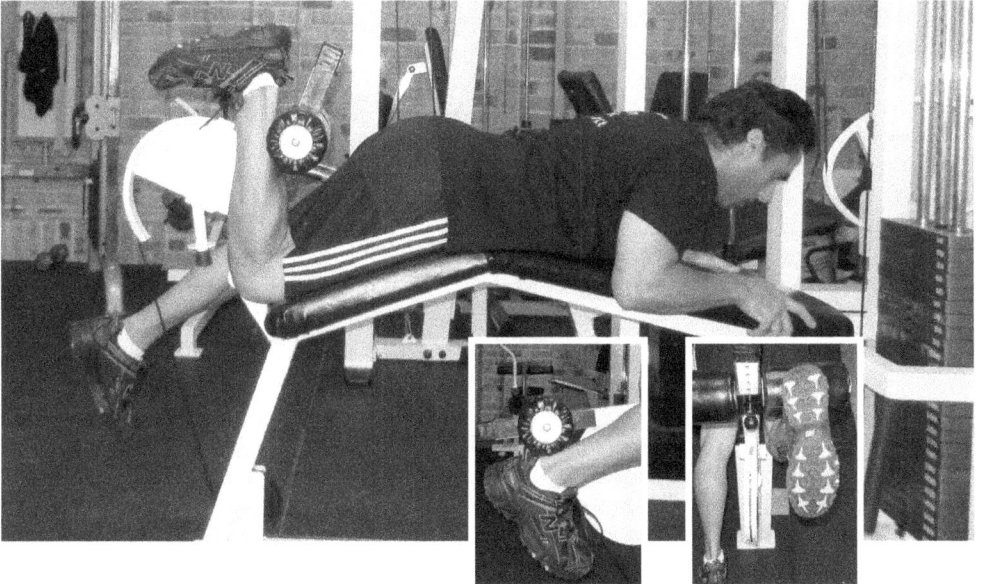

Dorsiflexed
(toes upward)

Neutral
(toes forward)

Prone: Superior – Medial Aspect

Start:

Lie prone, raise the opposing pelvis, abduct and medially rotate the working leg, invert and dorsiflex the foot, then flex the working leg at the knee joint at 90°.

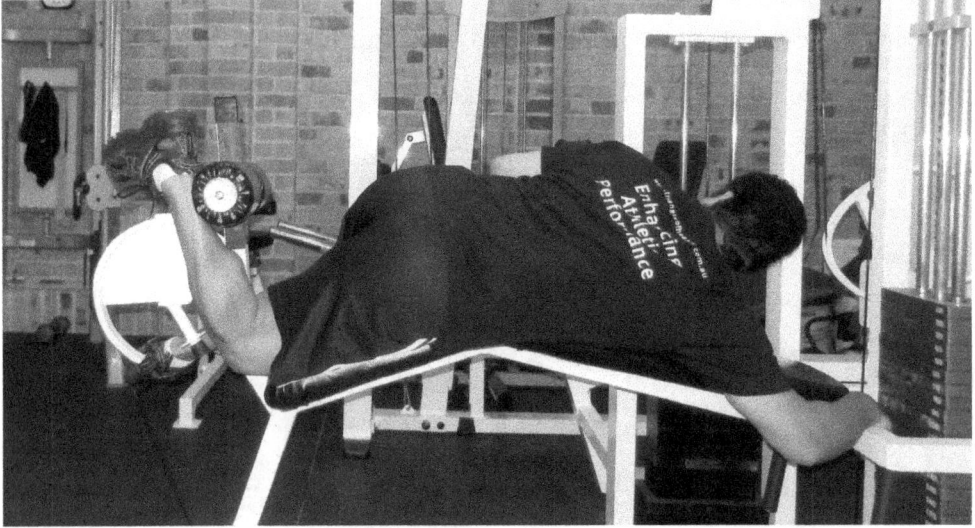

Finish:

Flex the lower half of the working leg at the knee joint, moving the foot in a medial direction to initial contact of calf and hamstring muscle in that leg.

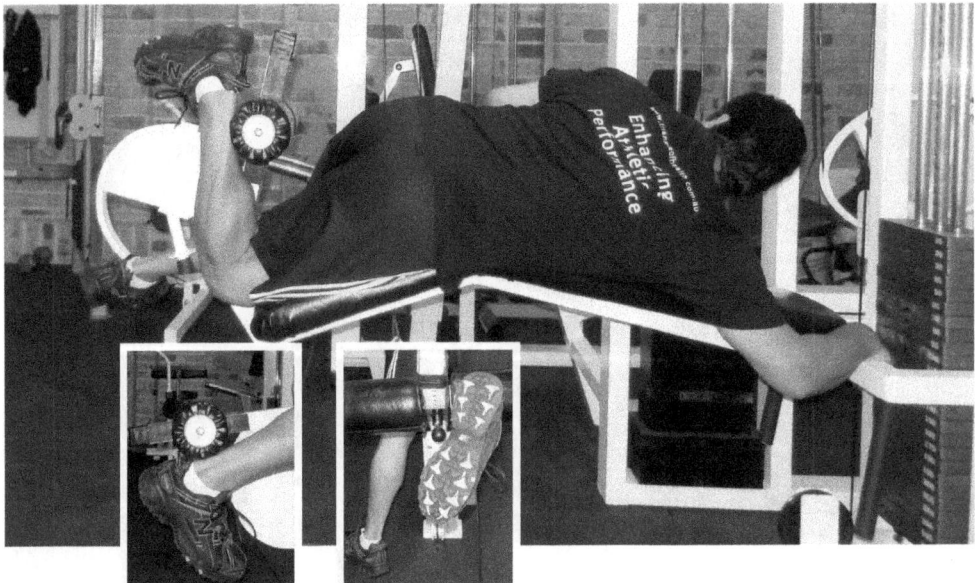

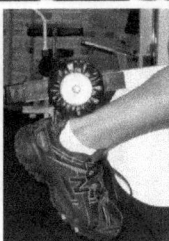

Dorsiflexed
(toes upward)

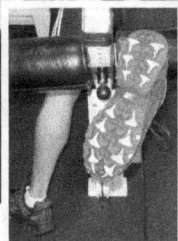

Inverted
(toes inward)

Prone: Inferior – Lateral Aspect

Start:

Lie prone, raise the pelvis, adduct and laterally rotate the working leg, evert and dorsiflex the foot, then flex the working leg at the knee joint below 90°.

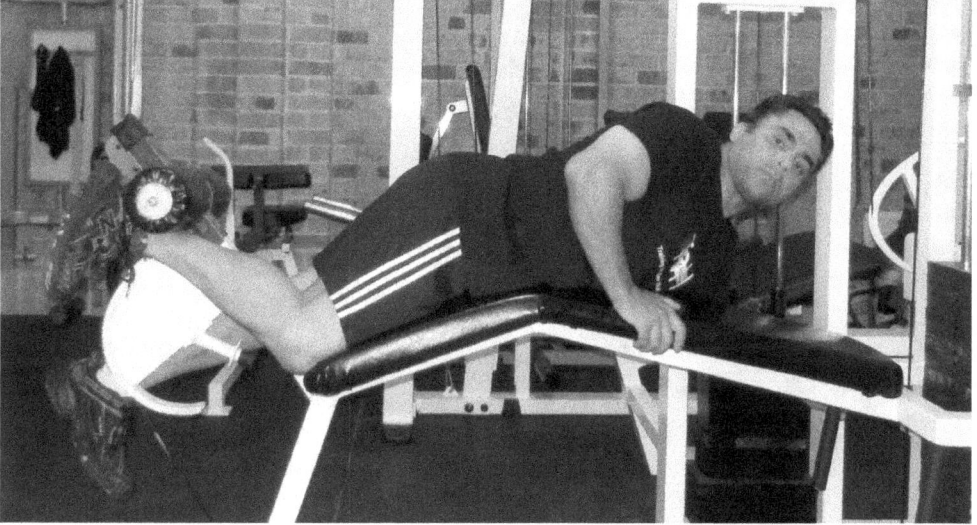

Finish:

Flex the lower half of the working leg at the knee joint, moving the foot in a lateral direction to 90°.

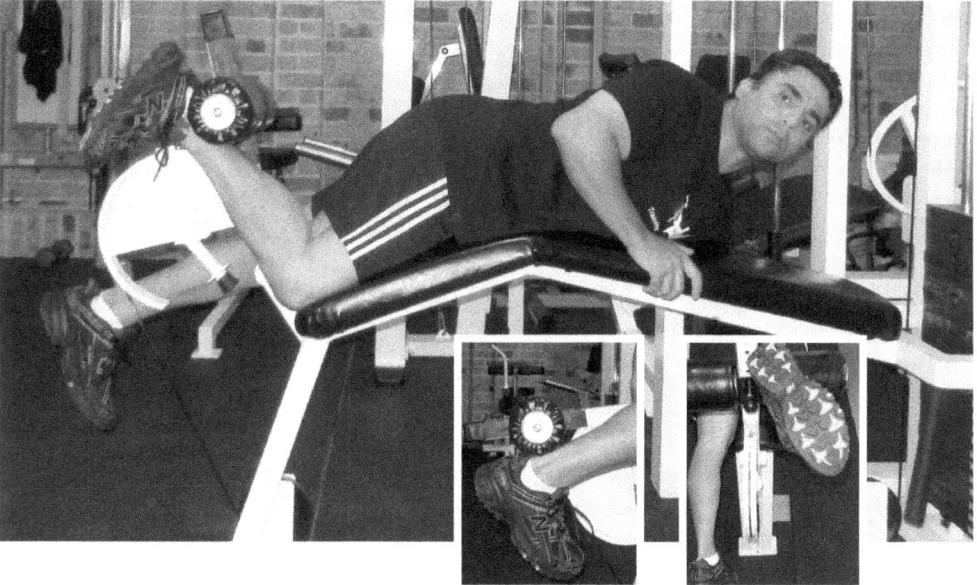

Dorsiflexed
(toes upward)

Everted
(toes outward)

Prone: Inferior – Middle Aspect

Start:

Lie prone, pelvis against the machine, the working leg aligned with the knee and the hip joint, the foot neutral and dorsiflexed, then flex the working leg at the knee joint below 90°.

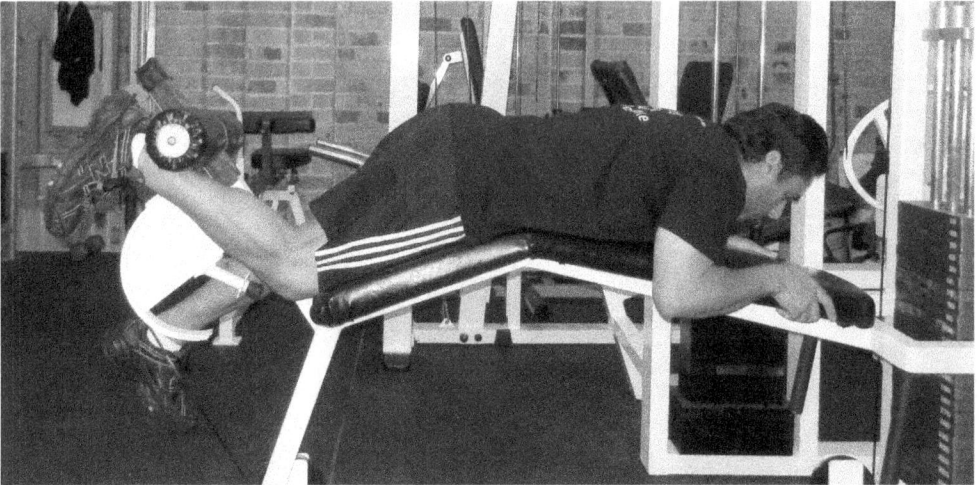

Finish:

Flex the lower half of the working leg at the knee joint, moving the foot in a forward direction to 90°.

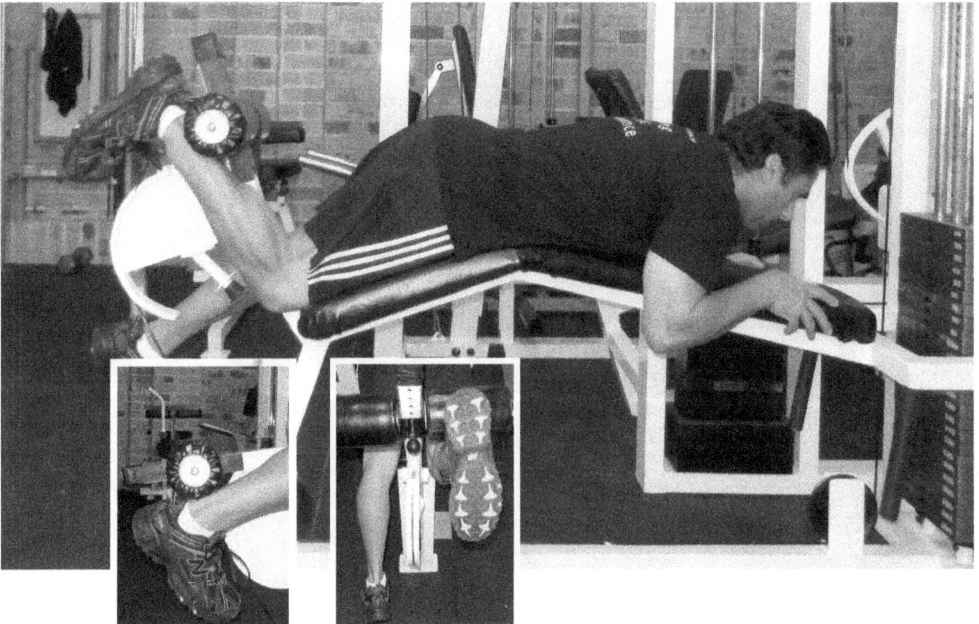

Dorsiflexed
(toes upward)

Neutral
(toes forward)

Prone: Inferior – Medial Aspect

Start:

Lie prone, raise the opposing pelvis, abduct and medially rotate the working leg, invert and dorsiflex the foot, then flex the working leg at the knee joint below 90°.

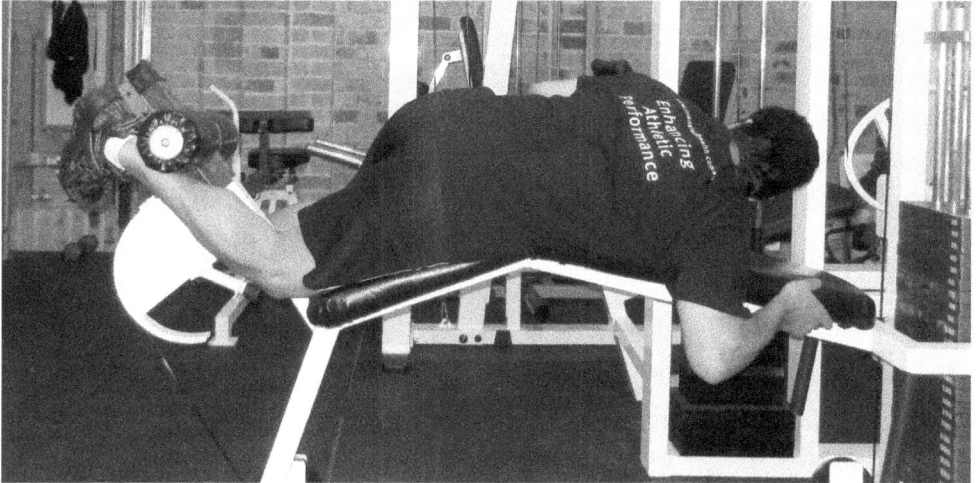

Finish:

Flex the lower half of the working leg at the knee joint, moving the foot in a medial direction to 90°.

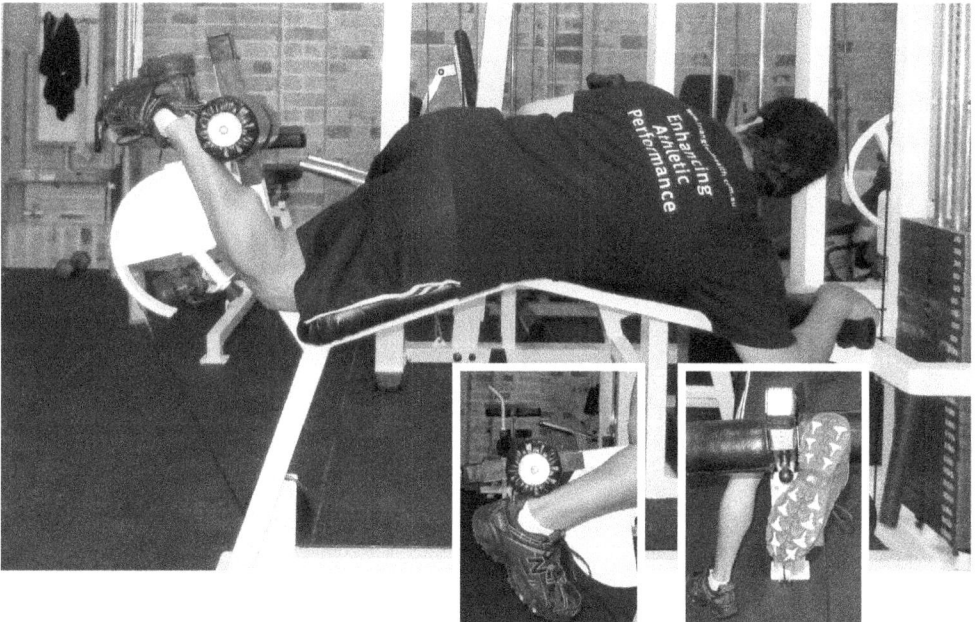

Dorsiflexed
(toes upward)

Inverted
(toes inward)

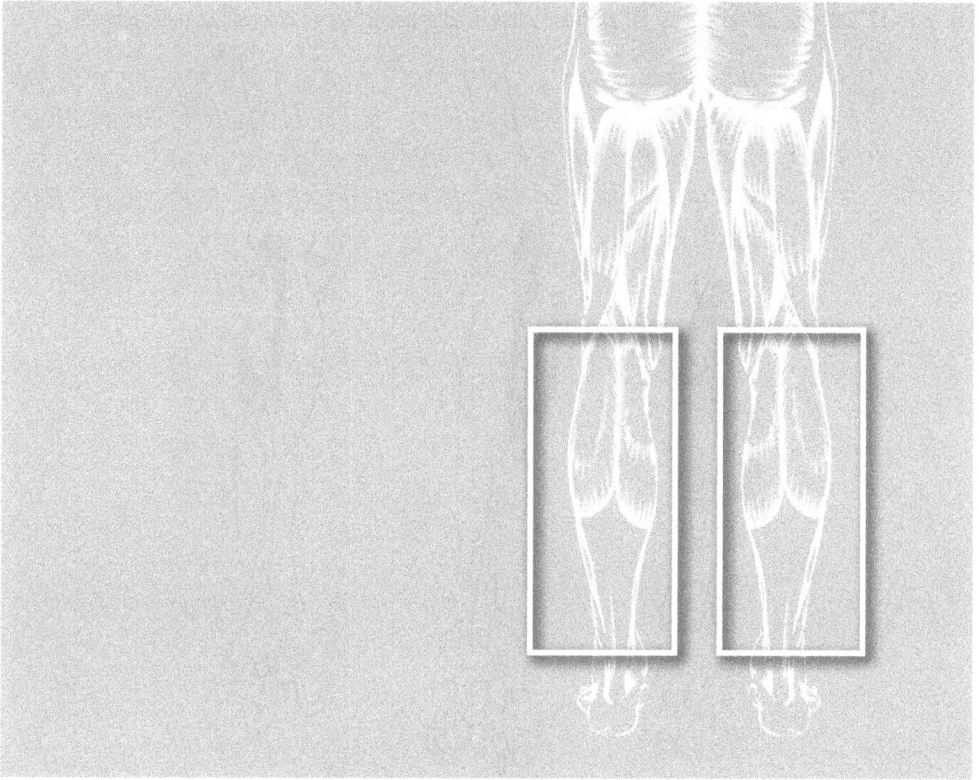

Calf Muscles Exercises

Gastrocnemius and Soleus

The gastrocnemius and soleus muscles combine to create what is commonly known as the calf, the main muscle of the lower leg, positioned to the rear.

The calf muscle is made up of two separate muscles:

- *soleus* – a horseshoe-shaped muscle positioned to the rear of the lower leg that functions to create plantar flexion (heel up, toes down) of the foot at the ankle joint

- *gastrocnemius* – a diamond-shaped muscle with two heads (lateral and medial) that sits on top of the soleus; it functions to create plantar flexion at the ankle joint and flexion of the lower leg at the knee joint.

Figure 13.12 Calf muscle (a) soleus (b) gastrocnemius (medial head) (c) gastrocnemius (lateral head)

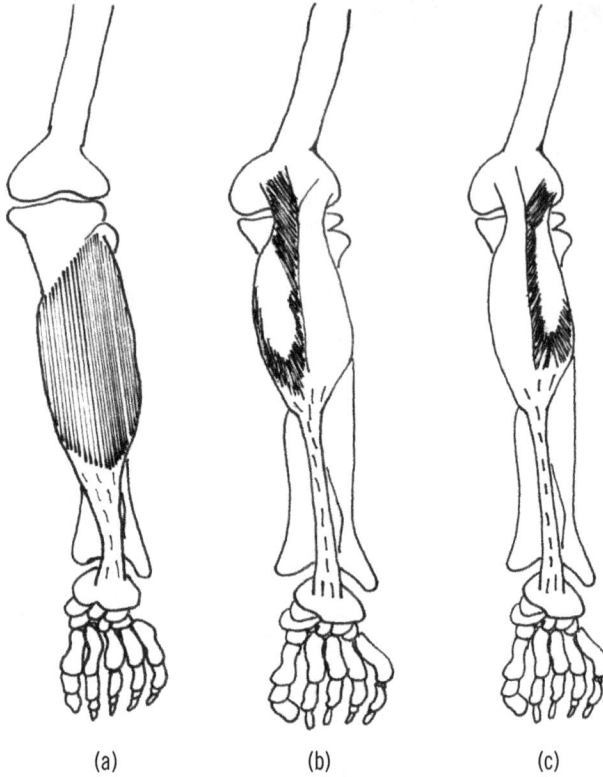

(a)   (b)   (c)

ORIGIN ATTACHMENT	INSERTION ATTACHMENT

Soleus
• **Tibia**
  (soleal line)
 	
• **Fibula**
  (upper two-thirds)
 	
• **Fibrous arch**
	• **Calcaneus**
	  (posterior)

Gastrocnemius (lateral head)
• **Femur**
  (lateral condyle)
	• **Calcaneus**
	  (posterior)

Gastrocnemius (medial head)
• **Femur**
  (medial condyle)
	• **Calcaneus**
	  (posterior)

Things to consider:

☑ Foot position for exercises for the calf muscles will be created via the hip, ankle and, in the case of the soleus, knee joints.

☑ Executing a calf raise with an extended leg will recruit both calf muscles.

☑ Executing a calf raise with the leg at a 90° angle will isolate the soleus, eliminating recruitment of the gastrocnemius muscle.

☑ During the calf curl exercise, it is imperative that the foot be maintained in a plantar flexed (heel up/ toes down) position, increasing gastrocnemius contraction, while decreasing hamstring recruitment.

☑ Everting the foot will assist in isolating the lateral aspect of the calf muscle; inverting it will isolate the medial.

☑ Allowing the heel of the foot to move past the alignment of the platform or structure in which calf raise exercises are carried out places the achilles tendon in a forced stretch position, increasing risk of injury.

LEG PRESS CALF RAISE (Gastrocnemius)

Seated: Inferior – Lateral Head

Start:

Align the working leg with the hip and knee joint and slightly evert the foot.

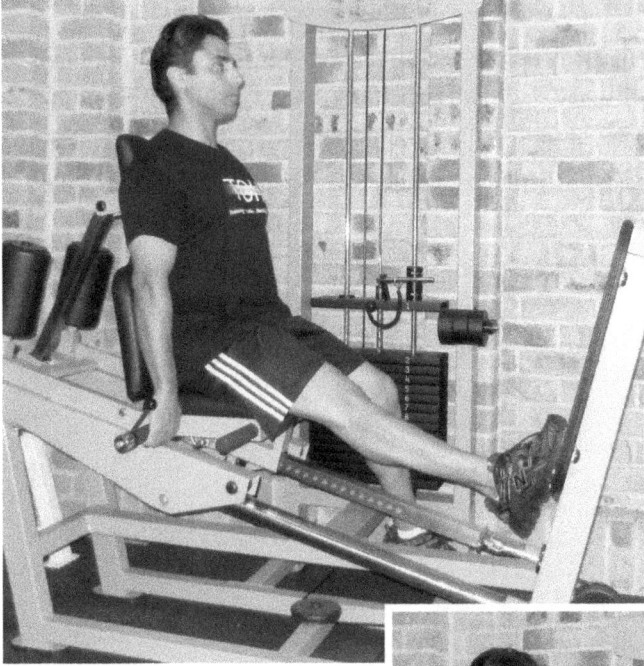

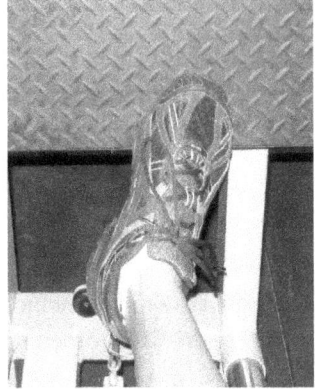

Everted
(toes outward)

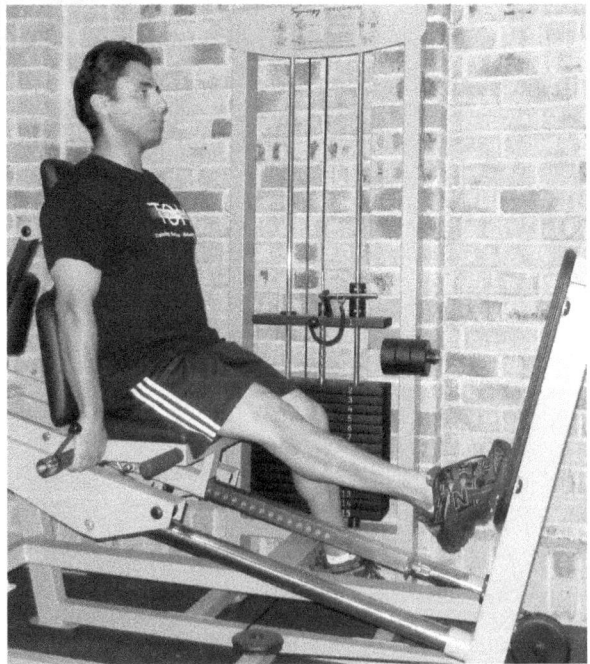

Finish:

Push against the footplate through the forefoot, raising the working heel in a medial direction to the initial point of stoppage.

(*Note:* Do not carry out exercise on your toes.)

Seated: Inferior – Middle Aspect

Start:

Align the working leg with the hip and knee joint, placing the foot in a neutral position.

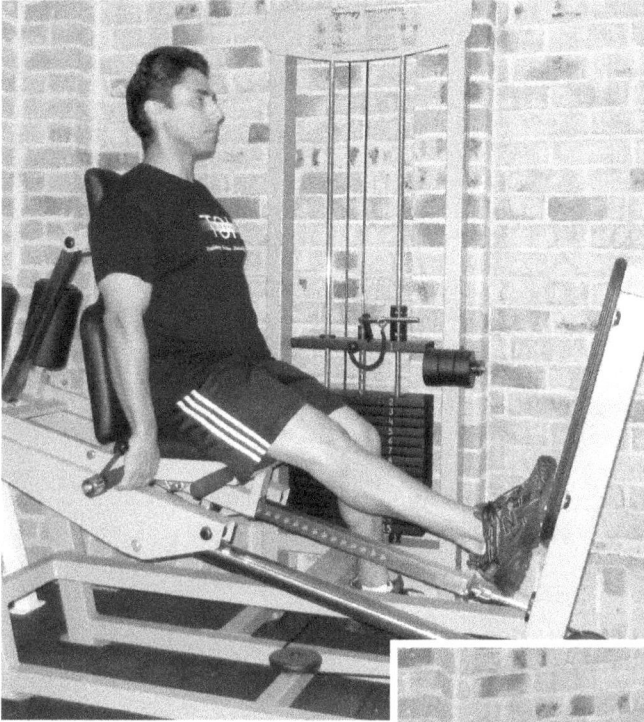

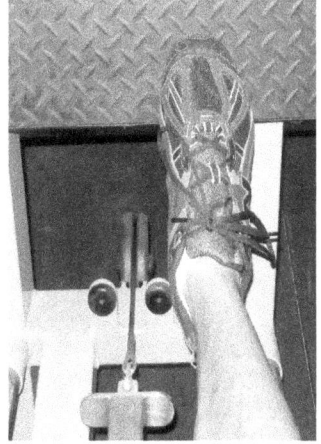

Neutral
(toes forward)

Finish:

Push against the footplate through the forefoot, raising the working heel in an upward direction to the initial point of stoppage.

(*Note:* Do not carry out exercise on your toes.)

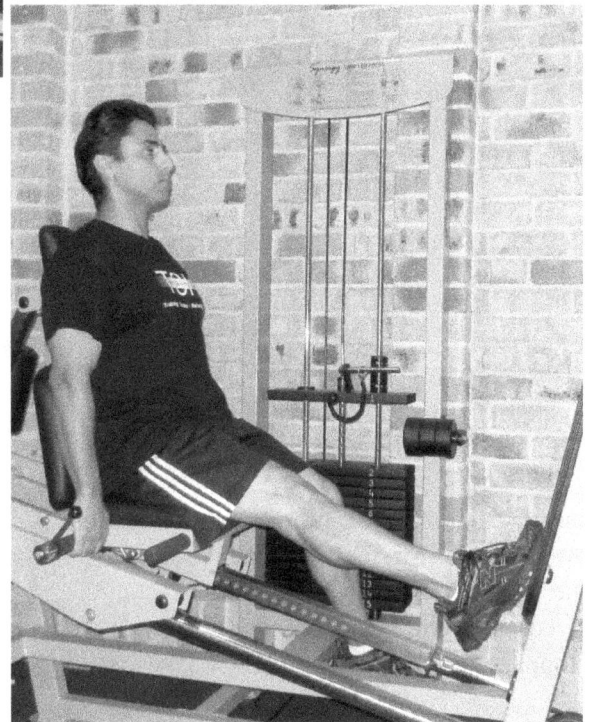

Seated: Inferior – Medial Head

Start:

Align the working leg with the hip and knee joint and slightly invert the foot.

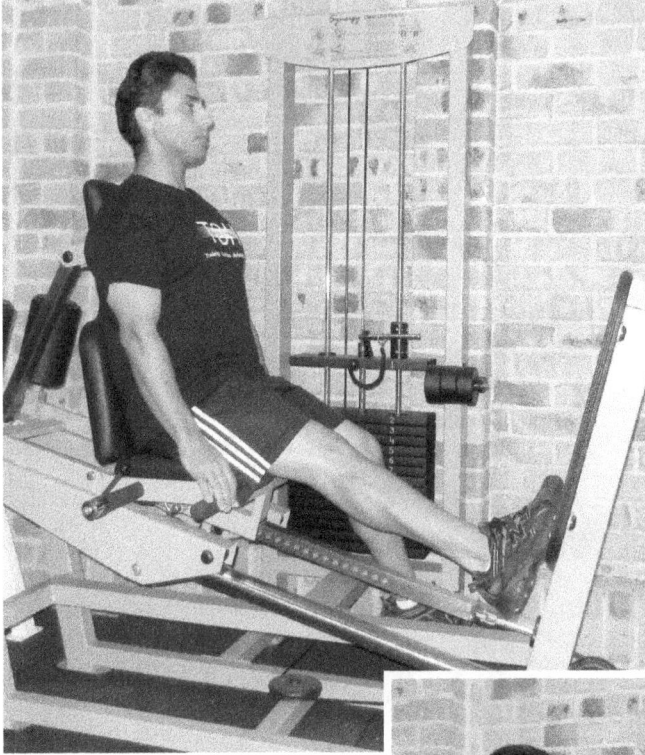

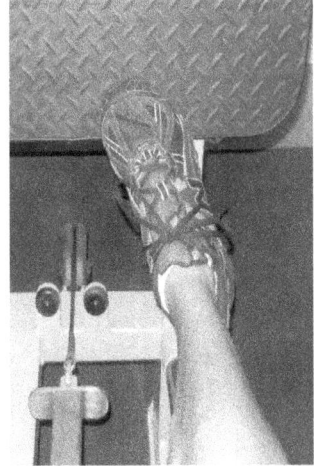

Inverted
(toes inward)

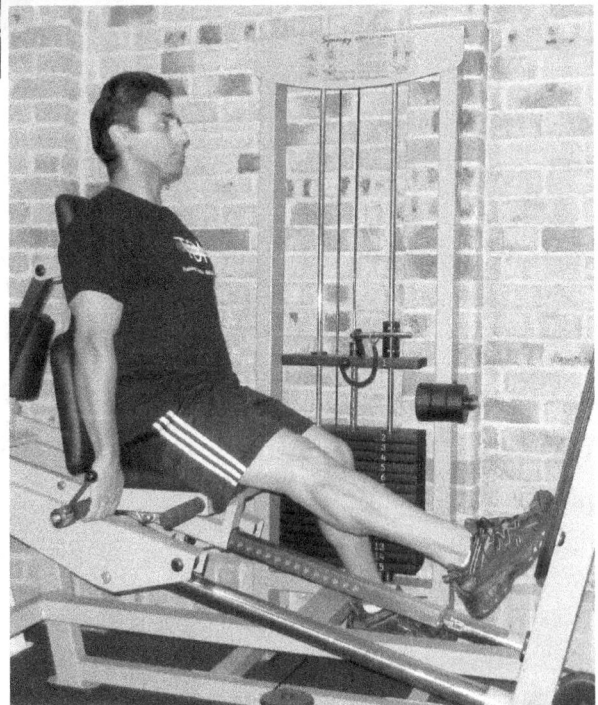

Finish:

Push against the footplate through the forefoot, raising the working heel in a lateral direction to the initial point of stoppage.

(*Note:* Do not carry out exercise on your toes.)

CALF LEG CURL (Gastrocnemius)

Prone: Superior – Lateral Head

Start:

Lie prone, with the working leg extended, with the pad positioned above the heel, then evert and plantar flex the foot.

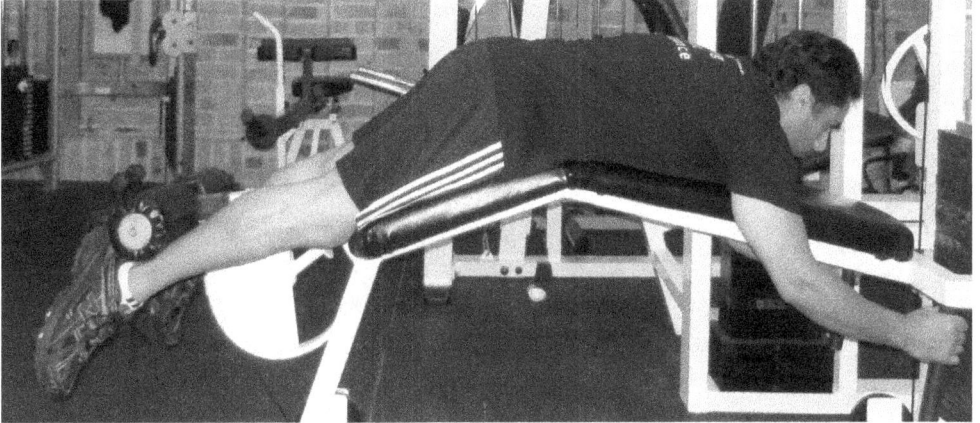

Finish:

Flex the working leg at the knee joint slightly, moving the foot in a lateral direction.

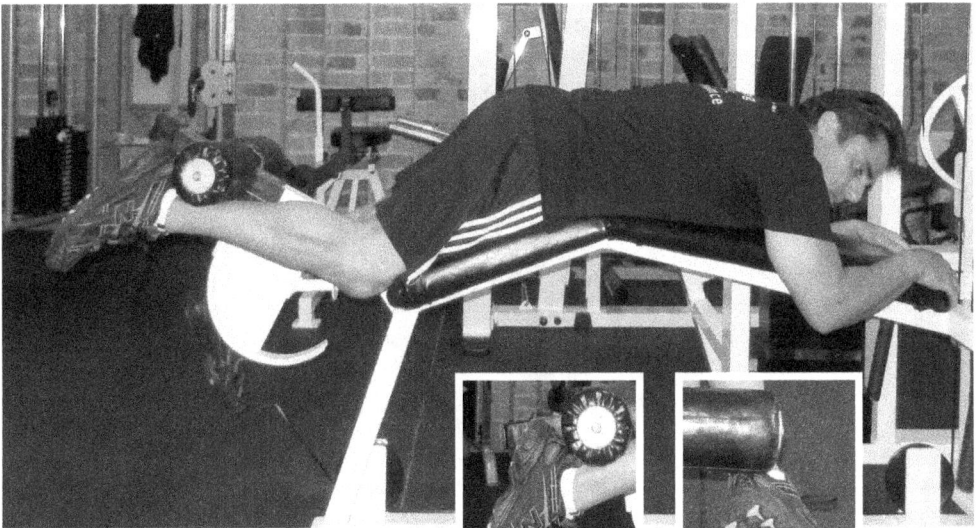

Plantar flexed
(heel upward)

Everted
(toes outward)

Prone: Superior – Middle Aspect

Start:

Lie prone, with the working leg extended, with the pad positioned above the heel, then place the foot in a neutral and plantar flexed position.

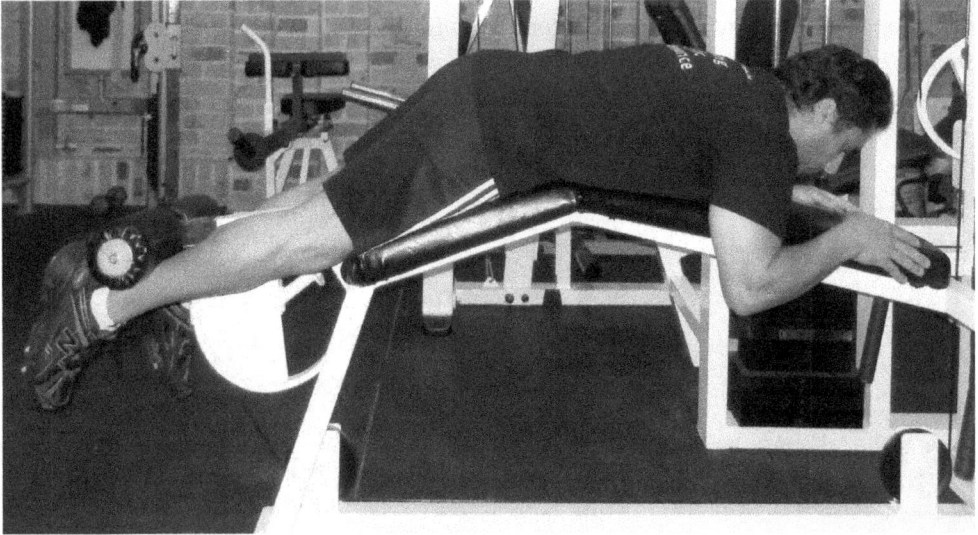

Finish:

Flex the working leg at the knee joint slightly, moving the foot in a forward direction.

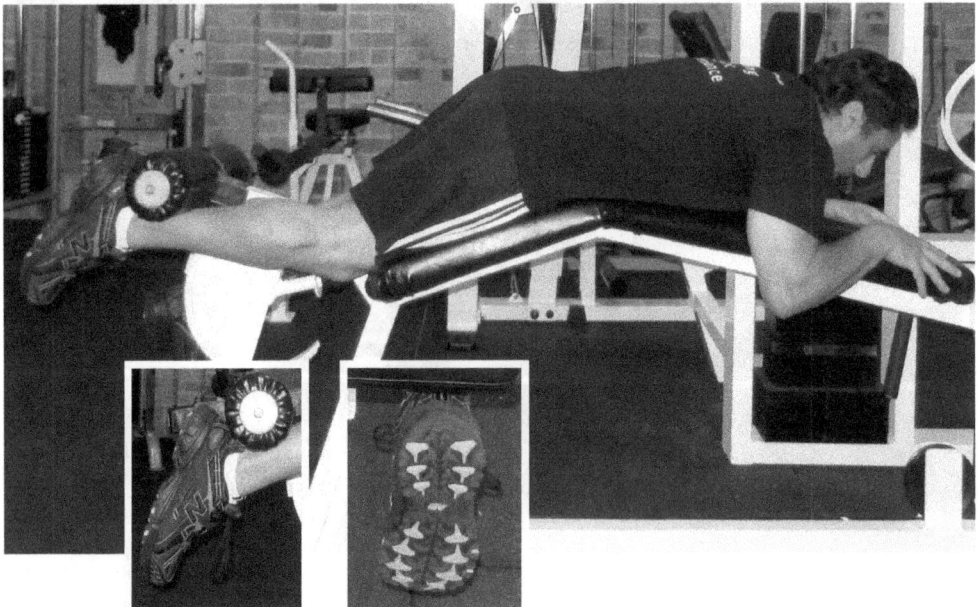

Plantar flexed
(heel upward)

Neutral
(toes forward)

Prone: Superior – Medial Head

Start:

Lie prone, with the working leg extended, with the pad positioned above the heel, then invert and plantar flex the foot.

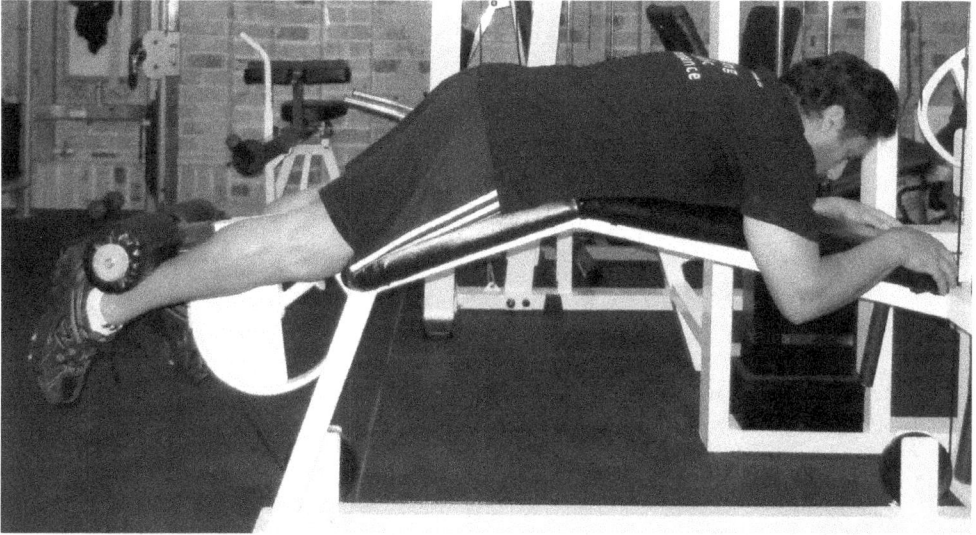

Finish:

Flex the working leg at the knee joint slightly, moving the foot in a medial direction.

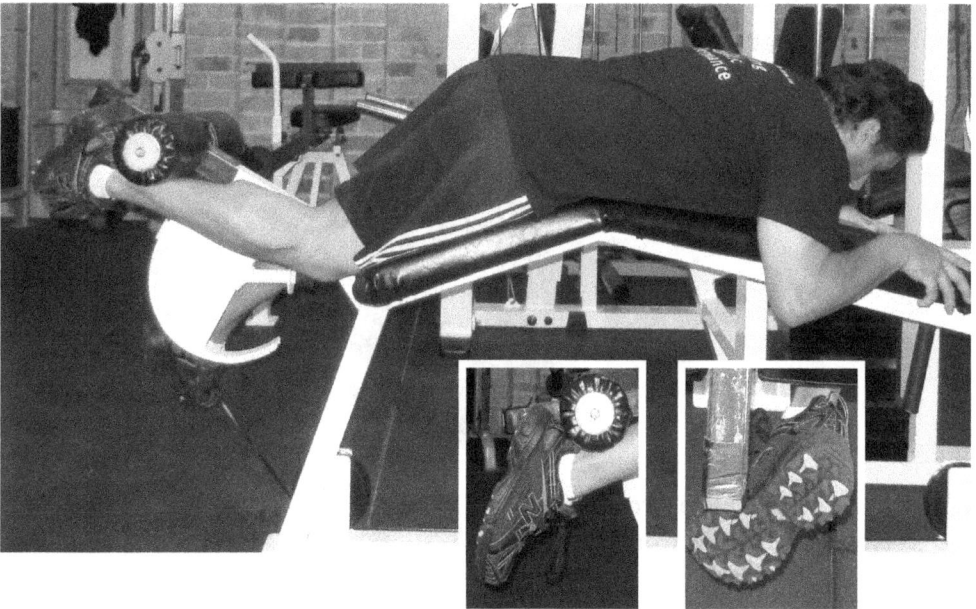

Plantar flexed
(heel upward)

Inverted
(toes inward)

CALF RAISE (Soleus)

Seated: Lateral Aspect

Start:

Sit, with the working leg at 90°, with the foot everted and aligned with the footplate.

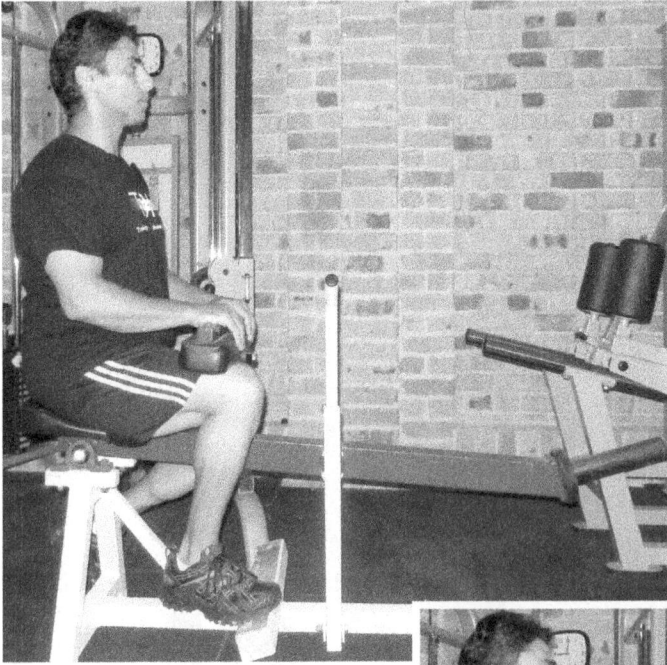

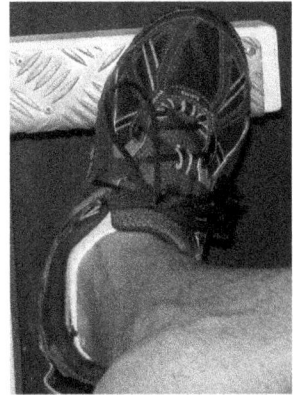

Everted
(toes outward)

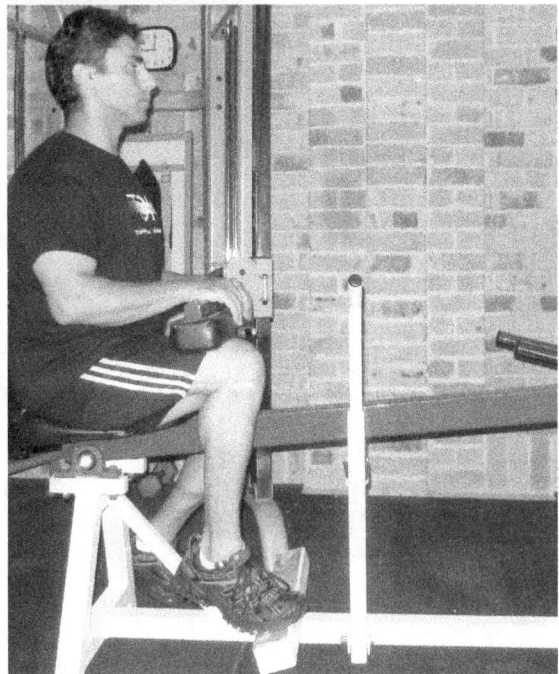

Finish:

Push against the footplate through the forefoot, raising the working heel in a medial direction to the initial point of stoppage.

(*Note:* Do not carry out exercise on your toes.)

Seated: Middle Aspect

Start:

Sit, with the working leg at 90°, with the foot neutral and aligned with the footplate.

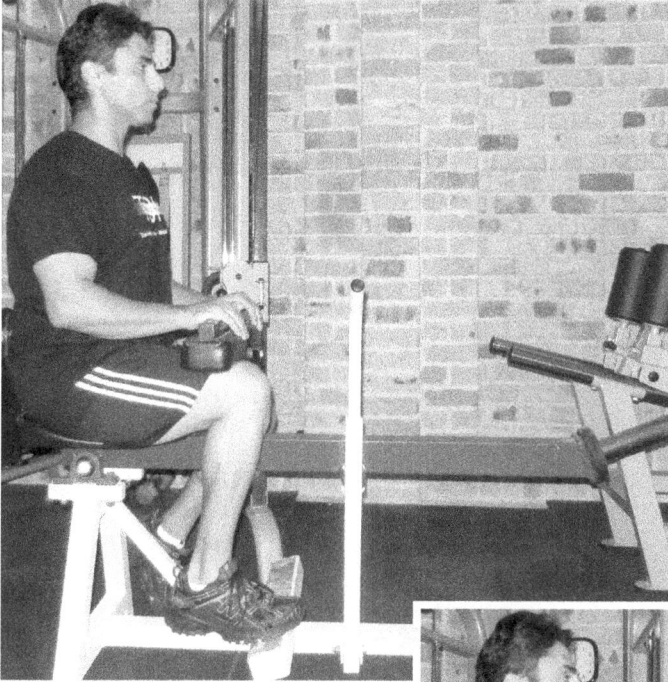

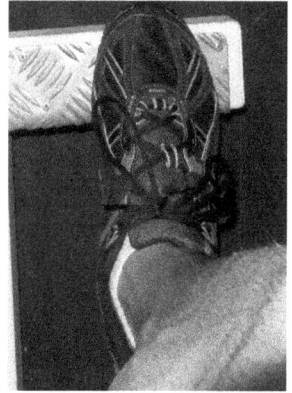

Neutral
(toes forward)

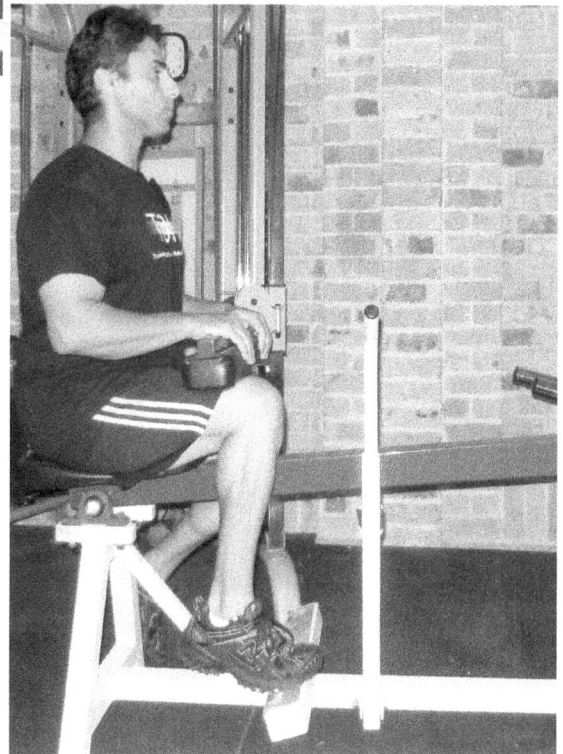

Finish:

Push against the footplate through the forefoot, raising the working heel in a forward direction to the initial point of stoppage.

(*Note:* Do not carry out exercise on your toes.)

Seated: Medial Aspect

Start:

Sit, with the working leg at 90°, with the foot inverted and aligned with the footplate.

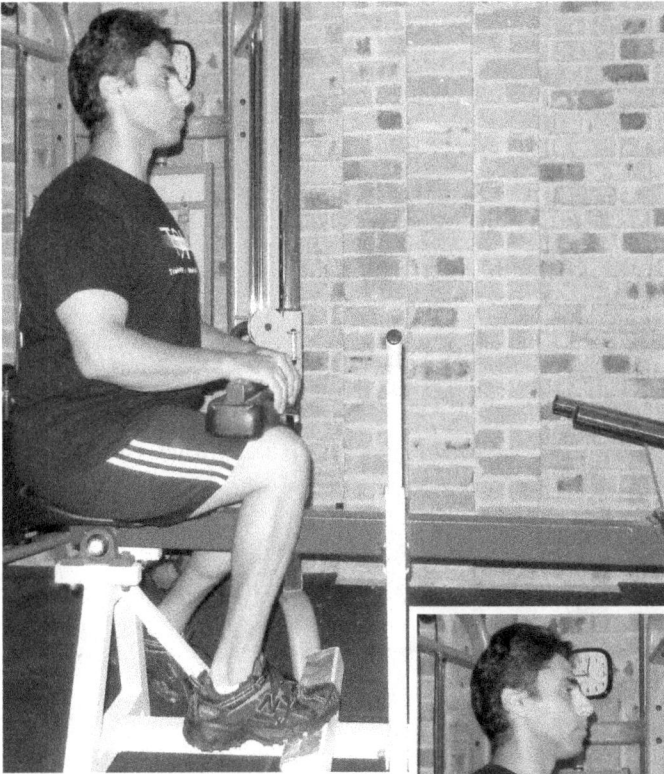

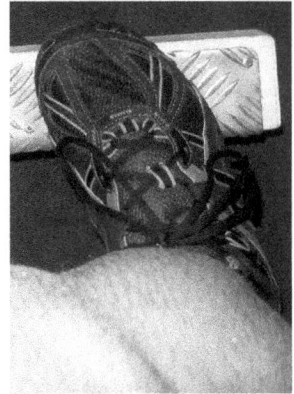

Inverted
(toes inward)

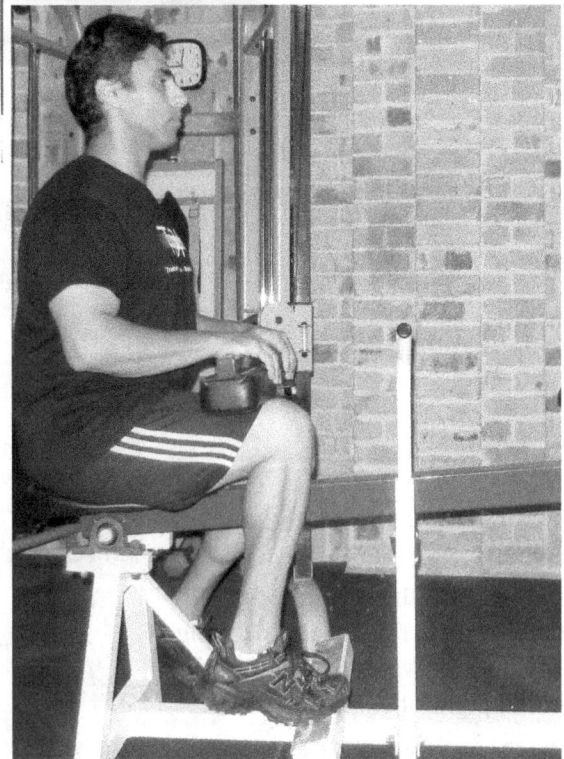

Finish:

Push against the footplate through the forefoot, raising the working heel in a lateral direction to the initial point of stoppage.

(*Note:* Do not carry out exercise on your toes.)

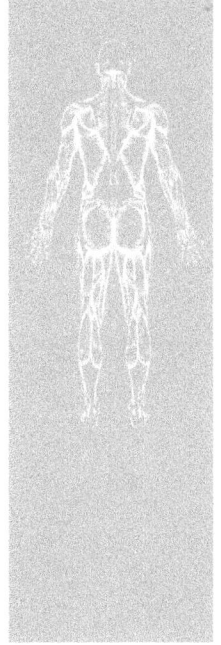

References

REFERENCES

SECTION ONE

Chapter 1

Ariel GB 1989. Biomechanics: scientific foundations of sports medicine. Toronto: B C Decker. p. 295.

Brainum J 2007. Warm up myths: bodybuilding for baby boomers. Iron Man Bodybuilding and Fitness (Australian edn) 14(10):36–44.

Burke P 2007. Train to gain (mature muscle) – reasons to lift. Iron Man Bodybuilding and Fitness (Australian edn) 14(9):26.

Fitnation 2008. Certificate IV in Fitness (SRF 40206). Advanced exercise programming and resistance training. Children and resistance training. p. 255.

Fitnation 2008. Certificate IV in Fitness (SRF 40206). Advanced exercise programming and resistance training. Injury prevention – Recovery. p. 210.

Fitnation 2008. Certificate IV in Fitness (SRF 40206). Advanced exercise programming and resistance training. Specifity principles – exercise prescription. p. 235.

Fitnation 2008. Certificate IV in Fitness (SRF 40206). Exercise for specific groups. Benefits of exercise postnatally. p. 37.

Fitnation 2008. Certificate IV in Fitness (SRF 40206). Exercise for specific groups. Safety standards for equipment. p. 321.

Johnson EM, Schmidt RR, Solomon EP, Davis PW 1985. Human anatomy. Part 2: Support and movement. Chapter 6: Muscle tissue and the muscular system. Philadelphia: Saunders College Publishing. p. 178.

Martin G 2013. Every cloud has a silver lining. The phrase finder.

Viewed 31 August 2012 <http://www.phrases.org.uk/meanings/every-cloud-has-a-silver-lining.html>.

Nosaka K 2007. Muscle damage and aging. Iron Man Bodybuilding and Fitness (Australian edn) 14(10):80.

University of Iowa n.d. Anaeorbic exercise: energy without oxygen. Viewed 25 August 2011 <http://www.uihealthcare.com/topics/exercisefitness/exer3098.html>.

Webster G (ed.) 2006. Encyclopedia of medical devices and instrumentation. Wiley: New York. Vol.1, 2nd edn. pp. 385–9.

Chapter 2

Fitnation 2008. Certificate IV in Fitness (SRF 40206). Advanced exercise programming and resistance training. Accommodating resistance. p. 163.

Fitnation 2008. Certificate IV in Fitness (SRF 40206). Advanced exercise programming and resistance training. Hypertrophy, strength–power, muscular endurance. pp. 151–3.

Fitnation 2008. Certificate IV in Fitness (SRF 40206). Advanced exercise programming and resistance training. Variable resistance. p. 164.

Hatfield FC 1989. Power, a scientific approach – advanced techniques for explosive strength and peak performance. Part I. Chapter 4: Elasticity and your stretch reflex. Chicago: Contemporary Books. pp. 24–7.

Hatfield FC 1989. Power, a scientific approach – advanced techniques for explosive strength and peak performance. Part I. Chapter 8: Ties that bind. Chicago: Contemporary Books. p. 53.

Hatfield FC 1989. Power, a scientific approach – advanced techniques for explosive strength and peak performance. Part II. Chapter 10: Getting started in a weight training program. Chicago: Contemporary Books. pp. 75–81.

Hatfield FC 1984. Bodybuilding, a scientific approach. Part II. Chapter14: The biomechanical principles behind the most commonly performed exercises. Chicago: Contemporary Books. p. 95.

McRobert S 2007. Train to gain (hardgainer): do you know your exercise categorisation? Iron Man Bodybuilding and Fitness (Australian edn) 14(9):30.

Chapter 3

Ariel, G 1996. Optimization of human performance for all ages. Speculations in Science and Technology 19:3–31.

Hatfield FC 1989. Power, a scientific approach – advanced techniques for explosive strength and peak performance. Part II. Chapter10: Getting started in a weight training program. Chicago: Contemporary Books, Inc. pp. 79–81.

Hatfield FC 1989. Bodybuilding, a scientific approach. Part II. Chapter 13: How high-tech equipment matches up to old fashioned hard work. Chicago: Contemporary Books. pp. 87–88,91.

Kennedy R 1983. Beef it: upping the muscle mass. Chapter 4: Machines or weights: questioning the superiority. New York: Sterling Publishing Co. Inc. p. 28.

LaPlaca J 2002. Cable system for exercise machine with multiple exercise stations. Patent references. Viewed 11 October 2007 < www.patentstorm.us/patents/6719673-description.html>.

Mastropaolo J 2001.
The maximum power stimulus
theory for muscle. CRS quarterly
37(4):13–220. Viewed 12 May
2007 <www.creationresearch.org/
crsq/articles/37/37_4/Muscle.htm>.

Thie JF 1973. Touch for health:
a practical guide to natural
health using acupressure touch
and massage. Muscle testing,
awareness. California:
DeVorss & Company. p. 12.

Webster G (ed.) 2006.
Encyclopedia of medical devices
and instrumentation. Wiley:
New York. Vol.1, 2nd edn.
pp. 385,397.

37(4):13–220. Viewed 12/05/07
<www.creationresearch.org/crsq/
articles/37/37_4/Muscle.htm>.

Thie JF 1973. Touch for health:
a practical guide to natural
health using acupressure touch
and massage. Muscle testing,
awareness. California: DeVorss
& Company. p. 11.

SECTION TWO

Introduction

Arial, GB 1983. Resistive training.
Clinics in Sports Medicine 2(1):57.

Ariel GB 1989. Biomechanics:
scientific foundations of sports
medicine. Toronto: B C Decker.
p. 290.

Johnson EM, Schmidt RR,
Solomon EP, Davis PW 1985.
Human anatomy. Part 2: Support
and movement. Chapter 6: Muscle
tissue and the muscular system.
Philadelphia: Saunders College
Publishing. p. 178.

Chapter 4

Ariel GB 1989. Biomechanics:
scientific foundations of sports
medicine. Toronto: B C Decker.
p. 276.

Finando D & Finando S 2005.
Trigger point therapy for myofacial
pain: the practice of informed
touch. Chapter 4: Diagnosis and
treatment. Rochester, Vermont:
Healing Arts Press. p. 25.

Gluckman G 1995. Muscle
balance and function development.
Solution4pain.com. Viewed
23 September 2007 <www.
solution4pain.com/articles/
mbf_development.html>.

Ruiz, M and Barber FA 2005.
Synchronicity in motion:
shoulder function depends on it.
Biomechanics 12(10):26.

The free dictionary. Viewed
25 August 2008 <http://www.
thefreedictionary.com/symmetry>.

Chapter 5

Hatfield FC 1989. Power, a
scientific approach – advanced
techniques for explosive strength
and peak performance. Part II.
Chapter10: Getting started in a
weight training program. Chicago:
Contemporary Books, Inc. p. 75.

Hatfield FC 1989. Power, a
scientific approach – advanced
techniques for explosive strength
and peak performance. Part
III. Chapter 27. Nerve injuries.
Chicago: Contemporary Books,
Inc. p. 210.

Health for Life 1985. Secrets of
advanced bodybuilding: a manual
of synergistic weight training for
the whole body. Planes of motion
(section). The rep (chapter). Los
Angeles: Health for Life. p. 10.

How Stuff Works. How shotguns
work. Viewed 15 February 2009
<http://science.howstuffworks.
com/shotgun1.htm>.

Kendall FP, McCreary EK,
Provance PG 1993.
Muscles – testing and function,
with posture and pain. 4th edn.
Chapter 1: Fundamental principles,
manual muscle testing. Baltimore:
Williams & Wilkins. p. 5.

Kraus Back and Neck Institute
n.d. Applying science to the art
of medicine. Viewed 20 May
2007 <www.lowback-pain.com/
krausbackandneckinstitute.medx.
htm>.

Mastropaolo J 2001. The
maximum power stimulus theory
for muscle. CRS quarterly

SECTION THREE

Chapter 6

Ariel G 1996. Optimization of
human performance for all ages.
Speculations in Science and
Technology 19(3–31):24.

Stone RJ & Stone JA 1990. Atlas
of the skeletal muscles. Chapter 6:
Muscles of the shoulder and arm
(deltoideus). Iowa: Wm. C. Brown
Publishers. p. 110.

Chapter 7

Fitnation 2008. Certificate IV
in Fitness (SRF 40206). Exercise
for specific groups. Age related
changes in postural stability. p. 145.

Kendall FP, McCreary EK,
Provance PG 1993.
Muscles – testing and function,
with posture and pain. 4th edn.
Chapter 2: Joint motions. Planes
(section). Baltimore: Williams &
Wilkins. p. 12.

Chapter 8

Fitnation 2008. Certificate IV in
Fitness (SRF 40206). Exercise
science and postural screening.
Shoulder joint. p. 47. Fitnation.

Gluckman G 1995. Muscle
balance and function development.
Solution4pain.com. Viewed
23 September 2007 <www.
solution4pain.com/articles/
mbf_development.html>.

Johnson EM, Schmidt RR,
Solomon EP, Davis PW 1985.

Human anatomy. Part 1:
Organisation of the body,
Chapter 1: The human body
– an introduction. Philadelphia:
Saunders College Publishing. p. 16.

Kendall FP, McCreary EK,
Provance PG 1993.
Muscles – testing and function,
with posture and pain. 4th
edn. Chapter 2: Joint motions.
Abduction, adduction, lateral
flexion and gliding (section).
Baltimore: Williams & Wilkins.
p. 14.

Mastropaolo J 2001.
The maximum power stimulus
theory for muscle. CRS quarterly
37(4):16.

Rodger W 2003. DVD: Dealing
with shoulder injuries. Brighton,
Victoria: Fitnation Pty Ltd.

Chapter 9

Arial, GB 1983. Resistive training.
Clinics in Sports Medicine 2(1):58.

Ariel G 1996. Optimization of
human performance for all ages.
Speculations in Science and
Technology 19(3–31):23.

Kennedy R & Weis DB 1989. Raw
muscle! – new hardcore techniques
for superhuman strength and
muscle mass. Chapter 6: The alpha
zone concept – Factor 2: Muscle
memory. Chicago: Contemporary
Books, Inc. p. 144.

Chapter 10

Brainum J 2006. Fast results:
how important is repetition
speed. Iron Man Bodybuilding
and Fitness (Australian edn)
13(10):20–1.

Fitnation 2008. Certificate IV in
Fitness (SRF 40206). Advanced
exercise programming and
resistance training. Sets. p. 149.

Maximal stimulation for
maximal growth 2007. Iron
Man Bodybuilding and Fitness
(Australian edn) 14(10):83–4.

The free dictionary. Viewed
7 August 2009 <http://www.
thefreedictionary.com/instincts>.

Chapter 11

Always S 1995. The rotators
and extensors of the hip:
gluteal musculature. Muscular
Development 32(7):47.

Always S 2007. Muscle form and
function: build brickyard thickness
in your lower chest with decline
dumbbell bench press. Muscular
Development 44(8):338.

Gluckman G 1995. Muscle
balance and function development.
Solution4pain.com. Viewed
23 September 2007 <www.
solution4pain.com/articles/
mbf_development.html>.

Hatfield FC 1989. Power, a
scientific approach – advanced
techniques for explosive strength
and peak performance. Part I.
Chapter 1: Strength training: a
fresh look at an age old topic.
Chicago: Contemporary Books,
Inc. p. 7.

Hatfield FC 1989. Power, a
scientific approach – advanced
techniques for explosive strength
and peak performance. Part II.
Chapter 10: Getting started in a
weight training program. Chicago:
Contemporary Books, Inc. p. 78.

Hatfield FC 1989. Power, a
scientific approach – advanced
techniques for explosive strength
and peak performance. Part
II. Chapter 10: How high-tech
equipment matches up to old
fashioned hard work. Chicago:
Contemporary Books, Inc. p. 91.

Kendall FP, McCreary EK,
Provance PG 1993.
Muscles – testing and function,
with posture and pain. 4th
edn. Chapter 2: Joint motions.
Abduction, adduction, lateral
flexion and gliding (section).
Baltimore: Williams & Wilkins.
p. 14.

Kennedy R 1983. Beef it: upping
the muscle mass – advanced
nutrition, shock-training strategies.
Chapter 4: Machines or weights:

questioning the superiority. New
York: Sterling Publishing Co. Inc.
p. 27.

SECTION FOUR

Introduction

Maximal stimulation for
maximal growth 2007. Iron
Man Bodybuilding and Fitness
(Australian edn) 14(10):83–4.

Chapter 12

Always S 2003. Muscle form
and function: huge rear shoulders
through bent over dumbbell lateral
raises. Muscular Development
40(12):268–70.

Always S 2003. Muscle form
and function: mammoth deltoid
mass with standing barbell
presses. Muscular Development
42(4):244–7.

Always S 2005. Muscle form
and function: barbell bench press
– king of upper body exercises.
Muscular Development 42(2):
232–4.

Fitnation 2008. Certificate IV in
Fitness (SRF 40206). Advanced
exercise programming and
resistance training. p. 14.

Kraus Back and Neck Institute
n.d. Applying science to the art
of medicine. Viewed 20 May
2007 < www.lowback-pain.com/
krausbackandneckinstitute.medx.
htm>.

Maximal stimulation for
maximal growth 2007. Iron
Man Bodybuilding and Fitness
(Australian edn) 14(10):86.

Riaucour CS 2003. DVD: Dealing
with back pain. Brighton, Victoria:
Fitnation Pty Ltd.

Rodger W 2003. DVD: Dealing
with shoulder injuries. Brighton,
Victoria: Fitnation Pty Ltd.

Chapter 13

Always S 1994. Triceps brachii: expanding the extensors of the elbow. Muscular Development 31(12):30–1,150,152,154.

Always S 1995. Anatomy and kinesiology of the upper and middle back. Muscular Development (32)5:38–9,224.

Always S 1995. Anatomy and kinesiology of the upper back: thickening the trapezius muscle. Muscular Development 32(4): 38–9,106,108.

Always S 1996. Posterior thigh: hamstrings of substance. Muscular Development 33(1):132–3,136–7.

Always S 2003. Muscle form and function: huge rear shoulders through bent over dumbbell lateral raises. Muscular Development 40(12):268–70.

Always S 2004. Muscle form and function: breaking the size barrier with one-legged seated calf raises. Muscular Development 41(1):262–4.

Always S 2005. Muscle form and function: chiseling lower leg diamonds with standing barbell calf raises. Muscular Development 42(10):265–7.

Always S 2005. Muscle form and function: growing gargantuan inner triceps with EZ French presses. Muscular Development 42(1):206–8.

Always S 2006. Muscle form and function: reverse cable preacher curls. Muscular Development 43(1):188–90.

Always S 2006. Muscle form and function: single leg extensions for igniting ripped thighs. Muscular Development 43(9):256–8.

Always S 2006. Muscle form and function: add some serious slabs of beef to your posterior thighs with seated leg curls. Muscular Development 43(11):194–6.

Always S 2008. Muscle form and function: reverse lagging back width (with stiff-arm pulldowns). Muscular Development 45(3): 298–302.

Fitnation 2008. Certificate IV in Fitness (SRF 40206). Advanced exercise programming and resistance training. Patello-femoral syndrome. p. 259.

Johnson EM, Schmidt RR, Solomon EP, Davis PW 1985. Human anatomy. Part 2: Support and movement. Chapter 6: Muscle tissue and the muscular system. Philadelphia: Saunders College Publishing. pp. 197,212.

Kendall FP, McCreary EK, Provance PG 1993. Muscles – testing and function, with posture and pain. 4th edn. Chapter 7: Lower extremity strength tests: medial hamstrings – semitendinosus and semimembranosus. Baltimore: Williams & Wilkins. pp. 208–9.

Rodger W 2003. DVD: Dealing with shoulder injuries. Brighton, Victoria: Fitnation Pty Ltd.

Shankman G 1991. The science of hamstring training: blue prints for a maximum gain, minimum risk program. Sports Medicine Foundation of America. Muscle and Fitness Magazine (Australian edn). p. 128.

Stone RJ & Stone JA 1990. Atlas of the skeletal muscles. Chapter 5: Muscles of the trunk (rectus abdominis). Iowa: Wm. C. Brown Publishers. p. 94.

Stone RJ & Stone JA 1990. Atlas of the skeletal muscles. Chapter 6: Muscles of the shoulder and arm (brachialis). Iowa: Wm. C. Brown Publishers. p. 103.

Stone RJ & Stone JA 1990. Atlas of the skeletal muscles. Chapter 6: Muscles of the shoulder and arm (brachioradialis). Iowa: Wm. C. Brown Publishers. p. 128.

Stone RJ & Stone JA 1990. Atlas of the skeletal muscles. Chapter 6:

Muscles of the shoulder and arm (deltoideus). Iowa: Wm. C. Brown Publishers. pp. 102,110.

Stone RJ & Stone JA 1990. Atlas of the skeletal muscles. Chapter 6: Muscles of the shoulder and arm (latissimus dorsi). Iowa: Wm. C. Brown Publishers. p. 105.

Stone RJ & Stone JA 1990. Atlas of the skeletal muscles. Chapter 6: Muscles of the shoulder and arm (pectoralis major). Iowa: Wm. C. Brown Publishers. p. 98.

Stone RJ & Stone JA 1990. Atlas of the skeletal muscles. Chapter 6: Muscles of the shoulder and arm (trapezius). Iowa: Wm. C. Brown Publishers. p. 104.

Stone RJ & Stone JA 1990. Atlas of the skeletal muscles. Chapter 6: Muscles of the shoulder and arm (triceps brachii). Iowa: Wm. C. Brown Publishers. p. 116.

Stone RJ & Stone JA 1990. Atlas of the skeletal muscles. Chapter 8: Muscles of the hip and thigh (biceps femoris, semitendinosus, semimembranosus). Iowa: Wm. C. Brown Publishers. pp. 171–3.

Stone RJ & Stone JA 1990. Atlas of the skeletal muscles. Chapter 8: Muscles of the hip and thigh: quadriceps (rectus femoris, vastus lateralis, vastus medialis, vastus intermedius). Iowa: Wm. C. Brown Publishers. pp. 166–9.

Stone RJ & Stone JA 1990. Atlas of the skeletal muscles. Chapter 9: Muscles of the leg and foot (gastrocnemius, soleus). Iowa: Wm. C. Brown Publishers. pp. 184–5.

The free dictionary. Viewed 17 January 2013 <http://encyclopedia. thefreedictionarycomLinea+alba+ %28abdomen %29>.

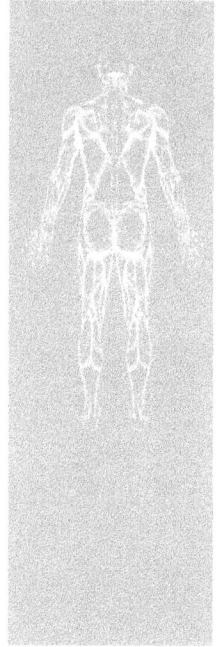

Glossary

GLOSSARY

A

Abdomen: section of the body between the chest and pelvis that encases various body organs such as the stomach, liver, intestines.

Abduct: *see* abduction.

Abduction: movement away from the mid-line of the body.

Abs: *see* rectus abdominis muscle.

Accelerated: increased speed.

Accelerated momentum: movement created in a rapid, swinging, uncontrolled manner by a prime moving muscle with the recruited help of other muscles.

Accommodating resistance training: a form of isokinetic exercise.

Acetabulum: cavity of the pelvis in which the head of the femur connects.

Achilles tendon: connective tissue that attaches the calf muscle to the heel.

Acromion process: outer end of the scapula situated near the lateral or outer aspect of the clavicle bone.

Action: *see* function.

Adduct: *see* adduction.

Adduction: movement towards the mid-line of the body.

Adductor: muscle that carries out an adduction movement.

Adjustable pulley: pulley that can be moved in various directions, up, down or across.

Aerobic: in the presence of oxygen; relating to energy production and exercise.

Aesthetic: relating to the physical shape and beauty of the human body.

Agility: executing body movement in a quick and nimble manner.

Anaerobic: in the absence of oxygen; relating to energy production and exercise.

Anatomy: structural, tangible components of the human body.

Angle: the position in which a muscle, joint, limb or body part is placed during an exercise.

Ankle joint: joint connecting the tibia and fibula bones with the talus bone.

Anterior: the front of a structure or in a forward direction.

Anterior dumbbell press: exercise that strengthens and conditions the anterior portion of the deltoid muscle with the arm in a flexed position.

Anterior dumbbell raise: exercise that strengthens and conditions the anterior portion of the deltoid muscle with the arm in an extended position.

Anterior inferior iliac spine: projecting bone of the ilium, proximal to the acetabulum.

Aponeurosis: thin sheet-like tissue that acts like a tendon in attaching muscles to bones.

Apparatus: device or piece of equipment.

Articulating cartilage: soft tissue present on the surface of two bones that form a joint.

Aspect: one of the four sections of a muscle: upper, lower, outer, inner.

Athletic performance: carrying out a physical activity in a sports-related field.

Atrophy: *see* muscle atrophy.

B

Ball and socket joint: synovial joint made up of one ball-like bone which fits into a shallow cavity of another bone structure; the joint can create a large range of movement known as circumduction.

Ballistic: movement created with explosive speed.

Barbell: exercise apparatus made up of a straight bar, generally made of metal, and discs known as weight plates that can be added to the bar to provide extra weight during exercise.

Barbell curl: biceps muscle exercise using a barbell.

Bent over dumbbell raise: exercise that strengthens and conditions the posterior portion of the deltoid muscle, with the arm in either a flexed or extended position.

Biceps brachii (*or* biceps) muscle: anterior portion of the upper arm comprising the short and long heads that create flexion of the forearm at the elbow joint, supination of the hand (due to the attachment at the radius bone) and weak flexion of the arm at the shoulder joint.

Biceps brachii muscle (long head): lateral aspect of the biceps muscle.

Biceps brachii muscle (short head): medial aspect of the biceps muscle.

Biceps femoris muscle: largest and most lateral aspect of the hamstring muscle, made up of two heads, short and long.

Biceps femoris muscle (long head): medial and larger aspect of the biceps femoris muscle involved in knee joint flexion and extension of the leg at the hip joint due to its pelvic attachment point.

Biceps femoris muscle (short head): lateral and smaller aspect of the biceps femoris muscle involved in knee joint flexion.

Bicipital aponeurosis: *see* aponeurosis.

Bicipital groove: deep groove at the upper end of the humerus bone.

Bilateral: refers to both sides of the body.

Bilateral sequence: executing a nominated number of repetitions on one side of the body without any rest, and then reciprocating on the other side to conclude a set.

Bilateral training: using a nominated prime moving muscle on both sides of the body to simultaneously execute an exercise.

Biomechanics: force and motion of the human body.

Biomechanically Correct (*or* BMC) Training System: resistance training system that functions on the premise of exercising one muscle on one side of the body at one time, catering to the natural biomechanics of the human body.

Blood vessels: tube structures that circulate blood around the body.

Bodybuilding: art of increasing muscle mass through resistance training exercise.

Bones: hard structural components that make up the skeleton of the human body.

Botox: toxic bacteria used as a commercial drug in the cosmetic industry to give an illusion of youthful appearance.

Brachialis muscle: upper arm muscle positioned beneath the biceps muscle, functioning to create flexion of the forearm at the elbow joint.

Brachioradialis muscle: lower arm muscle positioned on the forearm, functioning to create flexion of the forearm at the elbow joint.

Bursa sac: fluid-filled sac that stops or decreases friction between two structures, such as between bone and tendon, or between muscles near a joint.

Byproduct: side effect.

C

C7: seventh vertebra of the cervical spine.

Cable: metal wire enclosed in a plastic sheath placed around a pulley used to lift weight.

Cable-pulley adductor: exercise that strengthens and conditions the superior aspect of the triceps muscle with the arm in an abducted position.

Cable-pulley curl: exercise that strengthens and conditions the biceps muscle in various positions.

Cable-pulley extension: exercise that strengthens and conditions the triceps muscle in various positions.

Cable-pulley hammer curl: exercise that strengthens and conditions the brachioradialis muscle.

Cable-pulley lat pulldown: exercise that strengthens and conditions the latissimus dorsi muscle in two positions, with arm movement in a vertical position.

Cable-pulley leg flexion: exercise that strengthens and conditions the rectus femoris muscle.

Cable-pulley machine: resistance machine made up of pulley(s), cable(s), weight stack, guide rods and structural frame.

Cable-pulley reverse curl: exercise that strengthens and conditions the brachialis muscle.

Cable-pulley row: exercise that strengthens and conditions the latissimus dorsi muscle in two positions, with arm movement in a horizontal position.

Calcaneus: largest bone of the foot, commonly known as the heel.

Calf leg curl: exercise using a leg curl machine that strengthens and conditions the superior aspect of the gastrocnemius muscle in various positions.

Calf muscle: comprises two separate muscles, the gastrocnemius and soleus, positioned to the rear of the lower leg, and functioning to create plantar flexion of the foot at the ankle joint and flexion of the lower leg at the knee joint.

Calf raise: exercise that strengthens and conditions the soleus muscle.

Cam: spiral-like structure on a resistance machine used to change the load of a weight during an exercise.

Capsule: *see* synovial joint capsule.

Cardiorespiratory: relating to the heart and lungs.

Cartilage: connective tissue found in various areas of the body such as the ear, nose, rib cage and articulating surfaces of bones creating a joint.

Central nervous system: one half of the nervous system, comprising the brain and spinal cord, which controls the skeletal or voluntary muscles of the body by sending messages (impulses) from the brain to the muscles.

Centre of body mass: point where the three planes of the body – the sagittal, coronal and transverse planes – meet at right angles to each other.

Cervical spine: neck area of the spine made up of 7 individual vertebrae (C1 – C7).

Chemical reactions: metabolic processes in the body.

Chest: *see* pectoralis major.

Chin up: body-weight exercise that emphasises the biceps and latissimus dorsi muscles.

Chiropractic: therapy that employs manual adjustment of joints.

Chronic: constant, over a long period of time.

Clavicle: commonly known as the collar bone.

Clavicular head: origin of the pectoralis major muscle, attached to the clavicle bone.

Collagen: fibrous protein component found in bone and soft tissue structures such as cartilage, tendon and skin.

Collagen injection: cosmetic procedure used to improve skin appearance.

Compound exercise: any exercise or movement using multiple joints and muscles.

Concentric contraction: shortening phase of a muscle during its contraction, during which joint angle and muscle length decrease.

Conditioning: level of training or function.

Condyle: outward curved shape of a knuckle shaped bone.

Condyle (lateral): round projecting part of a bone situated laterally.

Condyle (medial): round projecting part of a bone situated medially.

Connective tissue: tissue structures such as ligaments, cartilage and tendons that connect, support and bind bones and muscles.

Constant resistance training: exercise in which the weight used remains constant and unchanged from the beginning to the end of a muscle contraction.

Continuous motion repetition: controlled and continuous speed of a muscle contraction.

Converging: movement by which two points come together.

Coracoid process: bent finger-shaped bone that projects from the front of the scapula.

Coronal plane: dimension or aspect of the body created when an imaginary vertical line passes from one side to the other, dividing the body into equal front and back sections.

Coronoid process: projecting part of the upper end of the ulna bone.

Cosmetic: relating to improvement of a person's physical appearance.

Costal: refers to rib bone(s).

Crest of pubic bone: area between the pubic tubercle and pubic symphisis of the pelvis.

Crunch: body-weight exercise that emphasises the abdominal muscle.

Curvilinear movement: movement created in a curved line.

D

Deadlift: powerlifting exercise in which a barbell is lifted from the floor using muscles of the back, hips and legs.

Decelerate: to reduce speed.

Deltoid tuberosity: projecting bone in the middle of the humerus.

Deltoideus muscle (*or* Deltoid muscle *or* Delt): shoulder muscle broken up into 3 different portions – anterior, middle and posterior – and functioning to create flexion and inward rotation, abduction, extension and outward rotation of the arm.

Diagnostic tool: means of identifying or determining something.

Digestive processes: processes involved in the breakdown of consumed products such as food.

Direction: the plane in which movement occurs.

Diverging: movement by which two points move away from each other.

Dorsiflex: *see* dorsiflexion.

Dorsiflexion: movement of the foot in which the heel moves downward and the toes move in an upward direction.

Dumbbell: miniature version of a barbell.

Dumbbell adductor: exercise that strengthens and conditions the superior aspect of the triceps muscle with the arm in an abducted position.

Dumbbell curl: exercise that strengthens and conditions the biceps muscle in various positions.

Dumbbell extension: exercise that strengthens and conditions the triceps muscle in various positions.

Dumbbell hammer curl: exercise that strengthens and conditions the brachioradialis muscle.

Dumbbell press: exercise that strengthens and conditions the anterior portion of the deltoid muscle.

Dumbbell reverse curl: exercise that strengthens and conditions the brachialis muscle.

Dumbbell shrug: exercise that strengthens and conditions the trapezius muscle.

E

Eccentric contraction: lengthening phase of a muscle during its contraction, during which joint angle and muscle length increase.

Elastic: refers to the flexibility of a muscle.

Elbow joint: articulation of the humerus, radius and ulna bones.

Elbow joint extension: movement created at the elbow joint resulting in the lengthening of the forearm, increasing joint angle.

Elbow joint flexion: movement created at the elbow joint resulting in the shortening of the forearm, decreasing joint angle.

Endurance: measurement of force associated with aerobic exercise.

Erector spinae: superficial spinal muscles that help create stability and movement of the spine.

Evert (foot): rotation of the foot by which the toes point outward.

Explosive: refers to exercise carried out in a very fast manner.

Extension: movement in a backward direction.

Extensor: a muscle that carries movement in a backward direction.

External oblique muscle: abdominal muscle situated either side of the trunk.

External occipital protuberance: protruding small bone on the external surface of the occipital bone of the skull.

F

Fascia: sheet or band of fibrous tissue that envelopes, separates or binds soft tissue structures such as muscles.

Femur: thigh bone.

Femur head: upper round end of the femur that connects with the acetabulum to create the hip joint.

Fibrous arch: bow-like structure between the tibia and fibula bones.

Fibula: lower leg bone situated to the outer side of the tibia.

Fixed movement pattern: movement in which a path cannot be altered.

Flexibility: refers to the uninhibited movement of a muscle when placed in a lengthened position.

Flexion: movement in a forward direction.

Flexor: a muscle that carries out movement in a forward direction.

Force: energy produced for a muscle to move an object.

Forced repetition: repetition carried out with assistance.

Forefoot: front area of the foot, commonly known as the ball.

Fossa: shallow cavity relating to skeletal structures.

Free weight: piece of equipment or apparatus that provides a weight that is not fixed to any structure and moves freely.

Fulcrum: point at which movement occurs.

Full range of motion: complete distance travelled by a contracting muscle.

Function: the specific movement(s) a joint or contracting muscle creates.

G

Gastrocnemius muscle: one half of the calf muscle comprising two heads – lateral and medial – that sit on top of the soleus muscle.

Gluteals: hip muscles: gluteus maximus, gluteus medius and gluteus minimus.

Gluteal tuberosity: raised line at the top and back of the femur bone.

Glycogen: energy stored in muscles.

Golgi tendon organ: special organ located at the tendon of a muscle that functions as a load receptor, sending messages to the brain about tension created by a muscle. Acts as a safety mechanism for a skeletal muscle or tendon by inhibiting the raising of a weight, via relaxation of the muscle, when excessive tension or stretching of a tendon occurs.

Gravity: type of force or energy that creates resistance against objects on earth.

Greater trochanter: protruding bone on the top and outer part of the femur bone.

Greater tubercle: projecting lump, lateral to the head of the humerus.

Guide rod: steel pole along which weight plates move up and down.

H

Hammer strength machines: plate-loaded machines that cater to variable resistance training that is created through a fixed converging and diverging manner. The function of this machine is demonstrated by the movement of the arms (which carry out the exercise), which move apart and then come together as part of the exercise routine.

Hamstring muscle: posterior portion of the thigh, made up of the biceps femoris, semitendinosus and semimembranosus, and functioning to create flexion and slight medial rotation of the lower leg at the knee joint and extension of the leg at the hip joint.

Head (or Heads): the (or more than one) origin attachment of a muscle.

Head of femur: *see* femur head.

Head of humerus: *see* humeral head.

High intensity: maximum effort expended during exercise.

Hip joint: ball and socket joint created through the connection of the femur head (the ball) and the pelvic cavity known as the acetabulum (the socket).

Hormone production: production, by glands, of chemical substances that control and regulate various functions of the body.

Humeral head: ball-like structure at the superior end of the upper arm bone.

Humerus: upper arm bone.

Hydraulic machines: machines that cater to accommodating resistance training through a mechanism of fluid inside a cylinder that controls the speed of motion.

Hyper-extend: *see* hyper-extension.

Hyper-extension: extension beyond what is perceived as normal backward movement.

Hyper-flexion: flexion beyond what is perceived as normal forward movement.

Hyper-movement: any movement created by a muscle or joint that travels beyond a normal distance or alignment.

Hypertrophy: *see* muscle hypertrophy.

I

Iliac crest: outer edge of the thick upper border of the ilium.

Iliotibial tract: connective tissue fascia that covers the upper end of the thigh. The top part is positioned below the tensor fascia latea muscle, connecting to the lateral part of the hip joint capsule, while the bottom part attaches to the knuckle-shaped bone on the outside of the tibia, known as the lateral condyle.

Ilium: upper portion and largest of the three bones that make up the pelvic girdle.

Imbalance: uneven, lacking balance.

Inertia: Inertia has a specific meaning in physics. In the context of this book, inertia is the resistance point of motion.

Inferior aspect: lowermost fibres of a muscle.

Infraglenoid tubercle: bony lump situated below the scapula cavity that is the attachment site for the triceps long head.

Intensity: degree of exertion or effort during an exercise.

Intermuscular septum: connective tissue (fascia) partition that separates muscles.

Intertrochanteric line: spiral line located at the front top end of the femur.

Interveterbral disc: round, flat, disc-like structure that separates two vertebrae, and acting as a shock absorber for the spine.

Invert (foot): rotation of foot by which the toes point inward.

Ischial tuberosity: projecting part at the lower end of the ischium.

Ischium: lower section of the pelvic girdle.

Isokinetic: *see* isokinetic exercise.

Isokinetic exercise: exercise carried out at a constant speed of movement, executed on a specialty piece of equipment.

Isolation exercise: exercise carried out with a single joint action, with the goal of isolating a muscle.

Isometric muscle contraction: contraction of a muscle in the absence of joint movement.

Isotonic muscle contraction: muscle contraction broken up into concentric (shortening of muscle fibres) and eccentric (lengthening of muscle fibres) phase in which movement is created at a joint.

J

Jamming: hyper-movement of a joint in which the articulating bones push against each other in a forceful manner.

Joint: point where two bones connect.

K

Kinesiology: natural biofeedback therapy that diagnoses and treats imbalances of the body through muscle testing.

Knee cap: *see* patella.

Knee joint: connection of the tibia and fibula bones with the femur and patella.

Knee joint extension: movement created at the knee joint resulting in the lengthening of the lower leg.

Knee joint flexion: movement created at the knee joint resulting in the shortening of the lower leg.

Kyphosis: abnormal condition where the cervical spine moves forward and the thoracic spine moves or develops backward, creating a hunchback appearance.

L

Lateral: position furthest away from the mid-line of the body.

Lateral aspect: outermost fibres of a muscle.

Lateral (body): lying on the side of the body.

Lateral dumbbell raise: exercise that strengthens and conditions the middle portion of the deltoid muscle.

Lateral head: the origin attachment of a muscle, furthest from the mid-line of the body.

Lateral rotation: outward rotating movement from the mid-line of the body.

Lateral supracondylar line: *see* supracondylar line.

Lateral supracondylar ridge: *see* supracondylar ridge.

Latissimus dorsi muscle (*or* lat): shoulder muscle situated to the rear of the body, and functioning to create movements of extension, adduction and medial rotation of the arm while also maintaining the bottom angle of the scapula against the rib cage.

Leg extension: exercise that strengthens and conditions the quadricep muscle.

Leg press calf raise: exercise that strengthens and conditions the gastrocnemius, one of the calf muscles.

Lesser tubercle: projecting lump, medial to the head of the humerus bone.

Lethargy: lacking energy, a state of fatigue.

Leverage: *see* mechanical advantage.

Lever arm: metal arm on a lever machine used to move weight plates.

Lever machine: machine that caters to variable resistance training whereby weight is moved via a fulcrum and lever.

Lever system: system that moves weight via a lever arm and fulcrum.

Ligaments: soft fibrous bands of connective tissue that are generally positioned on the outside of a joint capsule which help to maintain the connection and stabilisation of two articulating bones.

Ligamentum nuchae: strong ligament in the neck region that functions to support the head.

Linea alba: line of connective tissue composed of collagen that runs down the abdominal wall, separating the rectus abdominis muscle left and right.

Linea aspera: raised line that runs down the back of the femur, bone.

Linear movement: movement in a straight line.

Liposuction: cosmetic procedure in which fat is removed from under the skin.

Load: some form of weight or resistance.

Lordosis: abnormal condition where the lumbar region of the spine develops forward, creating a concave appearance.

Lumbar spine: lower area of the spine between the thoracic spine and sacrum made up of 5 individual vertebrae (L1 – L5).

M

Machine: a device that allows the execution of exercise.

Machine leg curl: exercise that strengthens and conditions the hamstring muscle.

Machine leg extension: exercise that strengthens and conditions the quadricep muscle.

Massage: natural therapy that uses the hands, elbows or devices to manipulate soft tissue structures of the body for healing and relaxation purposes.

Mechanical advantage: placing the body and its various parts in a position(s) to achieve optimal power and strength advantage from a muscle's lifting a weight.

Medial: position closest to the mid-line of the body.

Medial aspect: innermost fibres of a muscle.

Medial condyle: *see* condyle (medial).

Medial head: the origin attachment of a muscle closest to the mid-line of the body.

Medial rotation: inward rotating movement to the mid-line of the body.

Membrane: pliable layer of tissue that covers, separates or connects regions, structures or organs of the body.

Middle: position between medial and lateral.

Mid-line: imaginary line that runs through the middle of the body separating it into equal halves.

Mitochondria: structural component of a muscle cell where energy sources such as fat and carbohydrates are burned to produce energy.

Momentum: movement of mass or object.

Motion: movement.

Motor neuron: communication cell of the nervous system that creates skeletal muscle contraction.

Motor unit: motor neuron and the skeletal muscle fibres it activates.

Movement pattern: natural path through which a contracting muscle, corresponding joint(s) and exercise equipment or apparatus move.

Multi-joint: use of more than one joint during an exercise.

Muscle: *see* muscular system.

Muscle atrophy: decrease of muscle size.

Muscle belly: middle component of a skeletal muscle.

Muscle contraction: shortening of muscle fibres.

Muscle fatigue: inability of a skeletal muscle to continue its contraction due to exhaustion.

Muscle fibres: substructures of a muscle.

Muscle force: energy relating to power, strength and endurance.

Muscle head: *see* head.

Muscle hypertrophy: increase of muscle size.

Muscle insertion: attachment point of a skeletal muscle to a bony structure that creates movement.

Muscle origin: attachment point of a skeletal muscle to a bony structure that does not allow movement.

Muscle spindles: muscle length receptors acting as a safety mechanism to prevent injury. Muscle spindles remain in a lengthened position, stopping a skeletal muscle from contracting or shortening if a resistance is too great or if the force of a muscle contraction is insufficient.

Muscular system: fleshy structural component of the body that creates movement, provides stability, is a site for energy storage, and that protects the body and components (such as the organs).

Muscle tissue: the three types of tissue of which a muscle can be made: skeletal, smooth or cardiac.

Muscle tone: *see* tone.

Musculoskeletal: relating to the muscular and skeletal systems of the body.

N

Nautilus machine: a brand of exercise equipment that allows variable resistance exercise through a device known as a cam.

Neck: cervical region of the spine made up of various muscles between the head and shoulders that execute various movements.

Negative repetition: eccentric phase of an isotonic muscle contraction.

Nerve: *see* nerve fibres.

Nerve fibres (*or* nerve vessels): vessels of a neuron that receive and transmit impulses or information from inside and outside the body.

Nerve impingement: compression of a nerve fibre.

Nervous system: communication system of the human body made up of the central and peripheral nervous systems.

Neurons: communication cells of the human body.

Neutral foot: toes pointing straight ahead.

Neutral hand (thumb down): 90° between supine and prone, palm facing outward.

Neutral hand (thumb up): 90° between supine and prone, palm facing inward.

Nutritional supplements: nutrients such as vitamins, minerals, amino acids and herbs that are consumed as tablets, powders or injections.

O

Occipital bone: base of the head.

Olecranon process: projecting part of the ulna bone, the sharpest point of elbow.

Olympic barbell: bigger version of a standard barbell catering to large amounts of weight and commonly used during power and Olympic weight-lifting competitions.

One repetition maximum (1RM): maximum amount of weight used for a single repetition of an exercise.

Osteopathy: natural therapy that uses manipulation of bones and muscles as a means of treating health issues relating to the human body.

P

Palpation: using the hands to touch or feel.

Patella: small bone positioned at the front of the knee joint commonly known as the kneecap.

Patellar ligament: section of the quadricep tendon that extends from the patella to the tibia (also referred to as the patella tendon).

Peak contraction: firmest point of a muscle contraction.

Pectoralis major muscle (or pec): chest muscle made up of the clavicular and sternocostal heads that function to adduct, flex and medially rotate the arm while also helping to maintain the arm and shoulder in a downward direction.

Pelvis: connection of the pelvic girdle and sacrum.

Pelvic girdle: bowl-shaped bones positioned at the bottom end of the spine and separated by the sacrum, which bear the weight of the upper body and allow attachment of the legs.

Perceived scale: individualised fictitious scale for measuring training intensity.

Peripheral nervous system: one-half of the nervous system, comprising the sensory receptors and peripheral nerves that connect the internal and external environment of the body with the central nervous system.

Physiology: function of the structural or physical components of the human body.

Physiotherapy: therapy that uses exercise and massage for rehabilitation purposes.

Pin-loaded machine: resistance machine where weight is increased or decreased by inserting a metal pin into the desired weight plate.

Plane: one of the three dimensional aspects of the human body: sagittal, coronal or transverse

Plantar flexed: *see* plantar flexion.

Plantar flexion: movement of the foot by which the heel moves upward and the toes in a downward direction.

Plastic surgery: invasive surgery where sagging skin, atrophied muscles and fat are cut, manipulated and removed.

Plate-loaded machine: resistance machine where weight is increased or decreased by placing weight plates.

Plyometric training: exercise carried out through an isotonic muscle contraction, with a focus on the eccentric muscle contraction and created in a rapid explosive fashion.

Point of inertia (or POI): exact point of resistance to motion; *see* inertia.

Portion: *see* aspect.

Posterior: the back of a structure or in a backward direction.

Power: measurement of force created through strength and speed.

Prime moving muscle: target or nominated working muscle.

Pronating: *see* pronation.

Pronation: moving into a prone position.

Prone (body): lying on the front of the body, facing in a downward direction.

Prone (hand): palm facing downward.

Psychology: therapy that focuses on the human mind and how it functions.

Pubic symphysis: fibrous cartilage that connects the two pubic bones.

Pubic tubercle: projecting bone on the lateral end of the pubic bone crest.

Pulley: round plastic or steel structure that guides and supports a cable.

Push-up: body weight exercise that emphasises the chest and triceps muscles.

Q

Quadricep muscle (or quad): biggest and strongest of the thigh muscles, located at the front of the thigh and made up of four different heads: vastus lateralis, vastus medialis, vastus intermedius and rectus femoris.

R

Radial tuberosity: projecting part on the top end of the radius bone.

Radio frequency ablation: invasive procedure in which high-frequency electrical currents are passed through an electrode, creating heat that destroys abnormal cells.

Radius: shorter outer bone of the two bones that make up the forearm closest to the thumb.

Range limiting device: device on a resistance machine that limits range of motion.

Range of motion (or ROM): distance travelled when a muscle contracts, creating movement of a limb or body part at a joint.

Receptor: specialised cell that detects changes that occur to the human body through sensory stimulation.

Rectus abdominis muscle: trunk muscle separated left and right mid-line of the body by the linea alba and functioning to create bending of the spine and compression of the abdominal area.

Rectus femoris: one of the four muscles that make up the quadricep, comprising the anterior and posterior heads, and positioned between the vastus lateralis and medialis above the intermedius muscle. It functions to extend the lower leg at the knee joint and flexes the leg at the hip joint.

Rectus femoris (anterior head): origin attachment closest to the mid-line of the body.

Rectus femoris (posterior head): origin attachment furthest from the mid-line of the body.

Rehabilitation: process of recovery, restoring the body to its normal function after injury or illness.

Repetition (*or* rep): single muscle contraction.

Repetitions: multiple muscle contractions.

Resistance exercise: *see* resistance training.

Resistance machine: machine that offers some form of weight resistance. It may function through various mechanisms or devices, with the weight generally moving and being guided by steel rod shafts. A machine can be either pin loaded (whereby the changing of weight in a stack of plates is carried out by placing a metal pin into the hole of a weight plate) or plate loaded (whereby weight plates or discs are placed onto an accommodating structure on the machine.)

Resistance training: form of exercise whereby a weight or load creates resistance for a contracting muscle.

Resistance training equipment: any apparatus that offers some form of resistance.

Respiratory: refers to the breathing system of the body (e.g. the lungs).

Rest: recovery period between sets and exercises.

Ribs: bones that insert into the thoracic vertebrae and sternum, creating what is commonly known as the rib cage.

Rotary movement: movement in a spinning or turning manner.

Rotator cuff muscles: four muscles – infraspinatus, teres minor, subscapularis and supraspinatus – that create external and internal rotation of the arm at the shoulder joint.

S

Sacrotuberous ligament: connective tissue ligament that runs posteriorly from the sacrum to the projecting bone; ischial tuberosity situated at the lower part of the ischium.

Sacrum: trianglular-shaped bone made up of 5 fused bones positioned at the base of the spine and attaching to each hip bone.

Saddle joint: saddle-shaped joint found only at the base of the thumb which creates circumduction (or circular movement).

Sagittal plane: a dimension or aspect of the body that is created when an imaginary vertical line passes from front to back dividing it into equal left and right sections.

Scapula: triangular-shaped bone commonly known as the shoulder blade, positioned against the ribs at the rear upper portion of the back and serving as an attachment site for various muscles.

Scapula spine: projecting bone to the rear of the scapula that divides it into top and bottom sections.

Sciatic nerve: nerve fibres that supply information related to feeling (sensory) and movement (motor) to and from the brain to the hamstrings and lower leg muscles. An impeded sciatic nerve will cause tingling or numbness in regions of the lower back, hips and back of the thigh.

Scoliosis: abnormal condition where the spinal column develops or moves laterally in the thoracic region.

Segment motion: contraction of a prime moving muscle in parts.

Semimembranosus: one of three muscles that make up the hamstring, which is part membrane, with the origin of attachment medial to the mid-line of the body.

Semi-prone (hand): palm of hand at a 45° downward angle.

Semi-supine (hand): palm of hand at a 45° upward angle.

Semitendinosus: one of three muscles that make up the hamstring which is part tendon, with the origin of attachment medial to the mid-line of the body.

Set: allocated number of repetitions.

Shape: structural appearance.

Short (*or* partial) range of motion: short distance travelled during a muscle contraction.

Shoulder capsule: synovial joint capsule of the shoulder.

Single joint: use of one joint to execute an exercise.

Sit-up: exercise that strengthens and conditions the rectus abdominis muscle.

Size: refers to dimension or how big something is.

Skeletal: refers to bones.

Skeletal muscle: muscle attached to the skeleton of the body, crossing a joint(s) that creates movement; also called a voluntary or striated muscle.

Skeletal system: bones that make up the skeleton of the human body.

Skull: bones that create the face and encase the brain.

Spinal alignment: when the vertebrae of the spine are in line with each other or in their correct position, creating postural balance.

Spinal cord: one-half of the central nervous system; is it a long cylindrical cord that extends from the brain, housed through the cavity of the spinal column, and tapers at the L2 vertebra. The function of the spinal cord is to transmit information to and from the brain through the nerve fibres (axons) – known as the ascending and descending tracts – via the connection of the peripheral nerves. Thirty-one (31) pairs of peripheral nerves exit from the spinal cord.

Spindles: *see* muscle spindles.

Spine: *see* vertebral column.

Spinous processes: backward projecting bone of a vertebra.

Soleal line: raised line at the upper, posterior surface of the tibia bone.

Soleus muscle: one of two muscles that make up the calf muscle; it sits beneath the gastrocnemius muscle.

Spotter: person who assists someone during training when necessary.

Static device: an immoveable object, apparatus or machine used to carry out isometric resistance training.

Static resistance training: exercise catering to isometric muscle contraction characterised by placing a muscle against an immovable apparatus followed by a gentle push or pull; this creates a muscle contraction minus joint movement.

Sternocostal head: origin of the pectoralis major muscle attached to the sternum, external oblique muscle and costal bones.

Sternum: structure commonly known as the breastbone in which the ribs connect at the front of the body, contributing to the formation of the rib cage.

Sticking point: *see* point of inertia.

Stirrup handle: handle used to execute exercises on a cable-pulley machine.

Strength: measurement of force.

Striated muscle: skeletal muscle composed of the proteins actin and myosin, components that allow the contraction of a muscle.

Structural: relating to structure, physical components.

Styloid process base: projecting bone, situated at the lower end of the radius bone.

Superficial: situated close to the skin of the human body.

Superior aspect: uppermost fibres of a skeletal muscle.

Supination: moving into a supine position.

Supine (body): lying on the back of the body, facing in an upward direction.

Supine (hand): palm of the hand facing upward.

Supple: flexible and limber.

Supracondylar line: line situated above a condyle or condyles; *see* condyle.

Supracondylar ridge: raised line situated above a condyle or condyles; *see* condyle.

Supraglenoid tubercle: bony lump on the top section of the scapula cavity.

Supraspinal ligament: fibrous cord that connects the cervical vertebra (C7) to the thoracic vertebra (T12).

Symmetry: balanced or equalised appearance of muscles on either side of the body in respect to their size, shape, position and function.

Synovial joint: freely moveable joint recognised by its cavity structure.

Synovial joint capsule: structure that can be likened to a balloon made up of fibrous tissue that is loose and flexible and which surrounds a synovial joint. The inner lining of the capsule has a synovial membrane which produces synovial fluid for the cartilage of the joint. The role of a capsule is to control and stabilise the joint and to supply nutrients via the synovial membrane and fluid.

T

T6: Sixth thoracic vertebra.

T7: Seventh thoracic vertebra.

T12: Twelfth thoracic vertebra.

Tendon: strong connective tissue composed of collagen, situated either end of a muscle that functions to connect it onto a skeletal structure of the body.

Therapeutic practitioner: individual who practises a form of natural therapy, assisting people with injuries and various ailments of the body.

Thoracic spine: middle area of spine between the cervical and lumbar made up of 12 individual vertebrae (T1 – T12).

Tibia: one of the two lower leg bones commonly known as the shin bone.

Tibial tuberosity: projecting bone at the top end and front of the tibia.

Tone: natural firmness or tension of a skeletal muscle when it is not contracting. A toned muscle should be supple, relaxed and elastic during palpation.

Traditional resistance training: exercise carried out in a bilateral fashion.

Transverse plane: dimension or aspect of the body that is created when an imaginary horizontal line passes through the body from the front to back or side to side, dividing it into equal top and bottom halves.

Trapezius muscle (*or* trap): shoulder muscle situated at the upper and middle portion of the back and divided into three sections: upper, middle and lower. The upper trap functions to elevate the lateral aspect of the scapula; the middle adducts the scapula; and the lower depresses the scapula, maintaining it against the ribs.

Triceps brachii (*or* triceps) muscle: back of the upper arm made up of three heads – lateral, long and medial – that function to extend the forearm at the elbow joint, while the long head also assists in the adduction of the arm when it is abducted at the shoulder joint.

Triceps muscle (lateral head): origin of attachment furthest away from the mid-line of the body.

Triceps muscle (long head): origin of attachment positioned between the lateral and medial heads.

Triceps muscle (medial head): origin of attachment closest to the mid-line of the body.

Trunk: section of the body minus the head and limbs, also known as the torso.

Tuberosity: projecting part of a bone that functions as the attachment site for soft tissue structures.

Tuberosity of ischium: *see* ischial tuberosity.

Tuberosity of tibia: *see* tibial tuberosity.

Tuberosity of ulna: *see* ulna tuberosity.

U

Ulna: one of two bones that make up the forearm, situated closest to the mid-line of the body.

Ulna tuberosity: projecting part situated at the top and front lower surface of the coronoid process.

Unilateral: refers to one side of the body.

Unilateral sequence: execution of all nominated repetitions and sets consecutively on one side of the body, then reciprocating on the other side.

Unilateral stance: position which has the left leg placed forward and right leg placed back, or vice versa, during an exercise.

Unilateral training: exercising a muscle on one side of the body at a time.

V

Variable resistance training: exercise in which the weight used increases or decreases in accordance with musculoskeletal leverage, and achieved via a mechanism such as a cam.

Vasti muscles: quadricep muscles vastus medialis, intermedius and lateralis.

Vastus intermedius: deepest of the four quadricep muscles, situated beneath the rectus femoris.

Vastus lateralis: most lateral of the four quadricep muscles.

Vastus medialis: most medial of the four quadricep muscles.

Vastus medialis oblique (*or* VMO): bottom portion of the vastus medialis muscle attached to the medial aspect of the kneecap that functions to carry out the last part of the lower leg extension by rotating the tibia on the femur.

Velocity: speed of movement.

Vertebrae: individual bones of different shapes and sizes that make up the spine; the singular is vertebra.

Vertebral column: main structure to which all other structures of the body attach, directly or indirectly, and commonly known as the spine. Made up of 26 individual bones, creating 5 sections – cervical, thoracic, lumbar, sacral and coccygeal – that are separated by disc-like structures that function as shock absorbers for the spine.

Vertical column: component of a cable-pulley machine that allows ascending or descending movement of a pulley(s).

Volume of work: amount of sets and repetitions carried out for an exercise.

Voluntary muscle contraction: contraction of a skeletal muscle that is consciously controlled.

W

Weight plate: individual weight that forms part of a weight stack, making up the resistance component of a machine.

Weight-bearing resistance exercise: exercise carried out with some form of apparatus that creates weighted resistance.

Weight stack: resistance component of a machine created by individual weight plates.

Working weight: resistance used by a prime moving muscle during an exercise.

X

Xiphoid process: the lower end of the sternum.

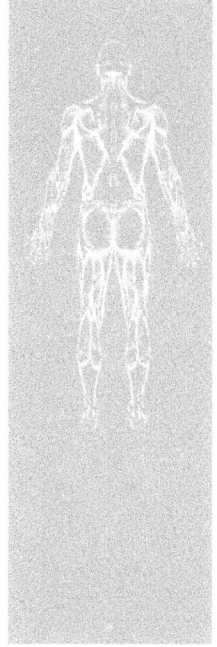

Index

INDEX

Feet
   muscle
      hamstring 177
      gastrocnemius, soleus 187
      quadricep 165
   position of 46
Femur
   attachment
      biceps femoris, short head 176
      vastus intermedius 164
      vastus lateralis 164
      vastus medialis 164
   condyle
      lateral 186
      medial 186
   definition 208
Fibrous arch 208
Fibula
   attachment
      biceps femoris, short head 176
      soleus 186
   definition 208
Fixed
   barbells 20
   capsule, shoulder joint 60
   equipment 21
   muscle, origin 58
Flexion
   definition 208
   dorsi 46
   exercise 172
   hyper 59
   muscle
      biceps 127
      brachialis 147–8
      brachioradialis 151
      gastrocnemius 185
      hamstring 176–7
      pectoralis major 100
      rectus femoris 172
      soleus 185
   plantar 46
Force
   definition 208
   gravity 63, 76
   lever machines, applied 21
   measurement of 11
   muscle
      generated 30, 44
Forced
   repetition, definition 208
Free weight
   definition 208
   equipment 20
   resistance, mechanism 14
Fulcrum
   definition 208
   machines, lever 21
Gastrocnemius
   definition 208
   exercises 188–193
   head
      lateral 186
      medial 186
   knee joint flexion, avoid 177
   muscle 185–6
Gluteal tuberosity
   definition 208
   femur 164
Golgi tendon organ 33, 208

Gravity
   definition 208
   inertia 63
   mechanical advantage 76
Greater trochanter
   definition 208
   femur 164
Guide rods
   resistance machine, component 21, 208
Hammer
   cable-pulley, curl 154
   dumbbell curl 153
   strength machines 22
Hamstring
   definition 209
   exercise 178–83
   muscle 175–6
Health and fitness
   facilities 6
   industry 19
Hip
   barbell deadlift 84–5
   barbell squat 82–3
   injuries to 88–9
   joint
      exercise 158, 160, 166–73, 179, 182, 187–90
      pain 77
      muscle, flexor 156
   width stance 47, 49
Hormone production
   definition 209
   resistance training, health benefits 8
Humeral head
   barbell military press, dangerous for 86
   capsule, shoulder joint 60
   definition 209
Humerus
   bicipital groove
      latissimus dorsi 120
      pectoralis major 100
   definition 209
   muscle
      brachialis 148
      brachioradialis 152
      deltoid 112
      latissimus dorsi 120
      triceps head, medial and lateral 138
Hydraulic machines
   ballistic movements, impossible with 22
   definition 209
   resistance training 22
Hyper-extension 209
   exercises, preventing 166–71
   lower arm 58
   quadricep exercises to prevent 165
   triceps exercises to prevent 138
   wrist joints 80
Hyper-flexion
   biceps 59
   definition 209
Hypertrophy
   definition 209
   resistance training, product of 11
Inertia
   avoiding 59
   benefits of exercising muscle in
   aspects 42
   definition 209
   dumbbell and cable-pulley machines 76

accommodating resistance training 15
  advantage of 76
  avoid POI, benefits for 64
  bilateral stance 47
  constant resistance training 14
  exercise, position/s for 47
  gravity 76
  machine, hydraulic 22
  unilateral resistance training 27, 29
  variable resistance training 15
Ligament(s)
  barbell military press, stretching 86
  barbell squat, pressure on 82
  definition 210
  injuries to 88–9
  ligamentum nuchae 108, 210
  shoulder, rotation 60
  supraspinal, 108
Ligamentum nuchae
  definition 210
  trapezius muscle108
Linea alba
  definition 210
  rectus abdominis 155
Linea aspera
  definition 210
  femur 164
Linear movement 210
Liposuction 8, 210
Load
  barbell squat, increase 83
  cam, change to 21
  definition 210
  exercise 10
  free weight 20
  inertia 63
Lower body exercises 161
Lumbar
  curvature, risk from barbell military press 86
  region 120
Machine
  definition 210
  dumbbell and cable-pulley, benefits of 76
  equipment 20–1
  exercises 104, 121-3, 133, 143, 146, 150, 154, 166, 172, 178, 188, 194
  pin-loaded 13
  plate-loaded 13
  resistance 213
Massage 7, 210
Mechanical advantage
  definition 210
  position, element 44
  range of motion, short 59
Middle
  definition 210
  muscle, fibres
    calf 189, 192, 195
    deltoid 39, 60, 111–14
    hamstring 179, 182
    latissimus dorsi 120, 123–6
    pectoralis major 102, 105
    trapezius 108
Mind–muscle connection 41
Mitochondria 8, 211
Motion
  aspect 52
  BMC Training System 56–7
  continuous, repetition 67

definition 211
gravity 76
inertia 42, 63
range of
  considerations influencing 60
  equipment 22, 56
  full 40
  ideal 58
  partial 59
segment 61, 70
speed 22
Motor
  neuron 30, 211
  unit 30
Movement
  accelerated momentum 29
  barbell curl 29
  barbell squat 17
  compound movement 79–89
  constant speed 15
  curvilinear 75–6
  definition 211
  directional 60
  equipment 13, 15–17, 21–2, 93
  full ROM muscle contraction 56, 59
  hyper 58, 67
  inertia 63
  joint 45–6
  linear 56–7
  motor units, 30
  natural 30, 51, 93
  negative effects of barbell 77
  pattern, components of 51–61
  range of motion 58–60
  rotational 47
  synovial joint 44, 52
  training
    bilateral resistance 31–2
    unilateral resistance 27, 30, 93
  unnatural 79–89
  weight of resistance 67
Muscle
  action 30
  aspects 40–2, 44, 60
  atrophy 8
  belly 60
  cell 8
  compound exercise 17, 79–89
  contraction
    hyper-flexion, abnormal 59
    incomplete 66
    partial 59
    peak 59
    single 56
  damage to 44, 58, 66
  exercise positions for 47–50
  fatigue 59, 67
  fibres 7, 30, 40–1, 44, 61, 66, 119
  force 11
  functions of 7
  head
    biceps, long, short 127–8
    definition 209
    gastrocnemius, lateral medial 185–6
    hamstring, long, short 175–6
    pectoralis major 99
    rectus abdominis 155
    quadricep, vastus lateralis, vastus intermedius, vastus medialis, rectus femoris (anterior,

ABOUT THE AUTHOR

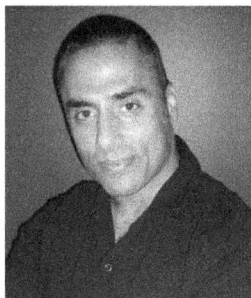

Darren Vartikian's passion for health and fitness began in 1988 with his burning ambition to become a professional bodybuilder. This led to an absorbing interest in the natural therapy kinesiology and, later, to a devotion to enhancing athletic performance. With diplomas in kinesiology and fitness, and registration as an exercise professional with Fitness Australia, Darren has combined formal education and practical experience over 26 years to accumulate a wealth of knowledge and insight into areas such as resistance training, nutrition and rehabilitation.

Darren's experience and skills – and his penchant for enhancing athletic performance – have created opportunities for him to work with both amateur and professional athletes in various sports. His driving commitment has been to guide and educate these athletes on how to achieve a competitive edge in a safe and efficient manner.

Always striving for perfection, Darren is never complacent, and is continuously asking questions and looking for answers.

Through his business, Triangle of Health (TOH) <website: www.triangleofhealth. com.au>, Darren has endeavoured to outline not only the services he provides but also his philosophies about enhancing athletic performance, health, fitness and general well-being.

His personal achievements include winning, in 1993, the prestigious IFBB Mr Australia (novice class) bodybuilding title at 22 years of age, following this up with runner-up winner in 1996.

Darren offers a simple philosophy he believes will help maintain longevity for those committed to reaping the benefits offered by his Biomechanically Correct Training System:

'Train smart; think about what you are doing.'

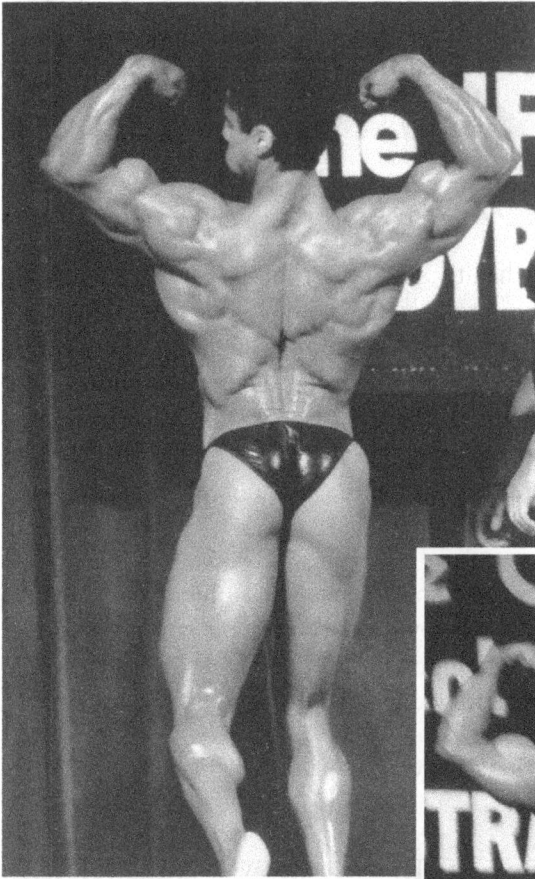

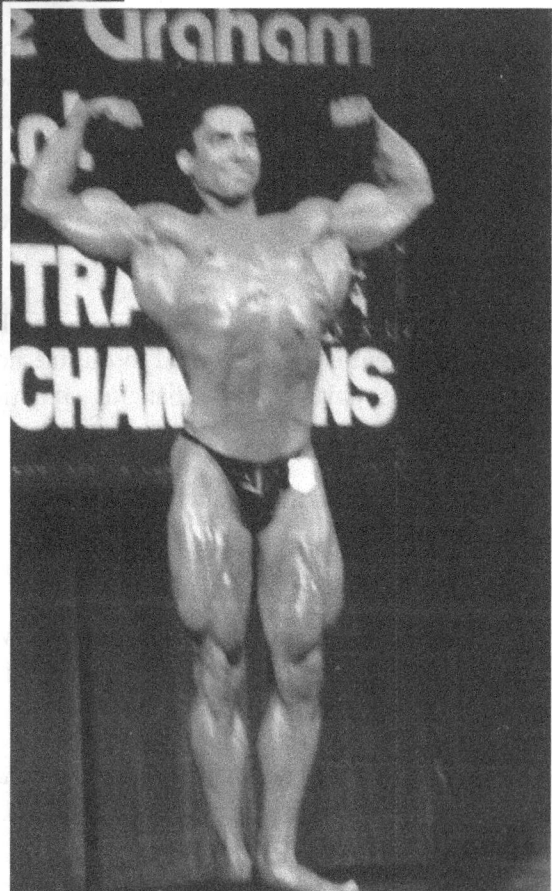

(*Photographs:* Darren Vartikian at 1993 IFBB
Mr Australia Championships.)